D0903206

HOMEOPATHIC THERAPEUTICS

Jacques Jouanny, MD
Jean-Bernard Crapanne, MD
Henry Dancer, MD
Jean-Louis Masson, MD

HOMEOPATHIC THERAPEUTICS

Possibilities in Acute Pathology

EDITIONS BOIRON

Same authors :

HOMEOPATHIC THERAPEUTICS :
Possibilities in Chronic Pathology

To avoid the awkwardness of "he/she", etc., the translators have used "he/him/his" throughout to refer to either gender, unless the context indicates otherwise.

Translated by Anne-Marie Cervera
and Tom Crawford

ISBN 978-2-85742-120-7

FORWARD

Homeopathic medicine is in its infancy in the United States, even though it has been used here for more than 150 years. The recent explosion of interest in homeopathy and other non-conventional modalities by the general public suggests that many of these therapies can no longer be considered "alternative" or outside the mainstream of medical practice. This increased public interest, coupled with current published scientific research in homeopathy and the growing realization that the cost of conventional high-tech medicine is out of control, has led a growing number of physicians to take a serious look at homeopathy.

In France, it is estimated that one-third of all physicians use homeopathy. Homeopathic medicines are available in all pharmacies and courses in homeopathy are taught in conventional medical and pharmacy schools. Studies done by the French Social Security system indicate considerable cost savings in patients treated with homeopathy. Most importantly, the French have developed a system of homeopathic education that is compatible with conventional medical thought.

This book offers U.S. physicians the opportunity to begin the practice of homeopathy for acute conditions, using the French methodology. After a brief explanation of homeopathic principles, the authors use a pathophysiologic approach to describe the modalities and clinical indications for a number of remedies commonly used for acute illnesses. This is followed by chapters on case-taking, prescribing of homeopathic remedies, and dosage and administration. The information on posology, or dosages, is a departure from what is commonly practiced in the U.S., since the French system relies on lower potency medications that are repeated more frequently and often used in combination with each other.

The second half of the book is devoted to the clinical application of homeopathy for common acute illnesses, using modern medical terminology rather than the more archaic terms found in many homeopathic texts. Organized by pathology and organ systems, this section gives indications for specific homeopathic medicines at various stages of illness. This section is invaluable for the busy clinician who wants a concise treatment guide for such ailments as influenza, bronchitis, teething problems, acute cystitis, skin eruptions, and trauma.

Homeopathic medicine is currently on the threshold of becoming more widely accepted and integrated into standard medical practice. It has been estimated by the French pharmacologist and homeopathic visionary Jean Boiron that 70% of all medical problems can be successfully treated with homeopathy, at a lower cost than conventional medicine and with no risk of side effects. Whether this vision will come to reality remains to be seen. Texts such as this, however, are essential to the process of bridging the gap between conventional and homeopathic medical thought and enabling physicians to successfully introduce homeopathy into their practices.

Jennifer Jacobs, MD, MPH

PART ONE

GENERAL POINTS

CHAPTER I

THE GENERAL PRINCIPLES AND METHODOLOGY OF HOMEOPATHY

Homeopathy is above all *a therapeutic method* which clinically applies *the phenomenon of similars* and which uses medicinal substances *in small or infinitesimal doses.*

For this definition to be comprehensible, the phenomenon of similars has to be explained.

THE PHENOMENON OF SIMILARS

This refers to the **observation of a physiological fact** as noted by Hippocrates and his school in the fifth century BC. It was observed, in fact, that there is often a **parallel between the toxic action of a substance and its therapeutic action**.

For example, white hellebore (*Veratrum album*) in toxic doses provokes intense diarrhea and vomiting accompanied by dehydration; the same white hellebore was used, in small doses, to treat Asian cholera epidemics which were particularly virulent at that time. This is a clear case of the parallel between the toxic action of a substance and its therapeutic action.

Similarly, cantharidin (*Cantharis*) in toxic doses provokes cystitis and hematuria; and yet cantharidin was used in small doses to treat urinary infections: a further example of the parallel between the toxic action of a substance and its therapeutic action.

Hence, in the oracular language of his time, Hippocrates said:

"The same things which cause a disease cure it".

In the centuries which followed, other physicians made similar observations though without drawing general conclusions.

It was not until the end of the eighteenth century, about 1790, that Christian Samuel Hahnemann, a German physician, who was also a chemist, a toxicologist, and an astute linguist, tried to verify **experimentally and scientifically** the Hippocratic conclusion which, after all, may simply have been an aphorism or a crude generalization of an accidental phenomenon.

So he proceeded in two stages:

- first of all, he collected the known toxicological data, and he studied the effects of the different substances of the pharmacopeia of his age, aconite, belladonna, arsenic, mercury, etc. on himself and his circle to find out which symptoms were caused by these products;

- secondly, he used these same substances, only this time as therapeutic agents, on sick people who presented similar symptoms to those he had obtained experimentally.

He then noticed that the phenomenon summarized by Hippocrates was borne out if small, or even infinitesimal, therapeutic doses were used:

- for example, if he gave ipecac to healthy people it provoked nausea, profuse vomiting, and hypersalivation. What was strange was that in spite of these intense digestive phenomena, the subjects' tongues remained clear or lightly coated and they were not thirsty;
- if he was dealing with patients suffering from dyspepsia, presenting symptoms of nausea and vomiting and the same accompanying group of signs (hypersalivation, clear tongue, absence of thirst), the administration of small doses of ipecac caused the disorders to disappear.

Similarly:

- if a healthy person is stung by a bee, a sudden reddish-pink edema appears at the site of the sting; the edema stings, burns, and the person instinctively tries to relieve it by applying something cold to it;
- with a patient showing a sudden edematous eruption that stings, burns, is relieved by applying something cold, but has a different cause (sunburn, urticaria caused by food, etc.), observation has proved that the taking of a microdose of bee venom reduces the symptoms. **Only a microdose of course**, since the patient is receiving a substance capable of producing under toxic conditions similar symptoms to those he is suffering from. Too strong a dose might on the other hand aggravate the pathologic symptoms.

It was thus **through observation and experimentation** that Hahnemann discovered **the necessity of small if not infinitesimal doses**.

And so, progressing from observation to observation and from experiment to experiment, Hahnemann realized that the Hippocratic hypothesis was true: **"medicinal substances are capable of curing symptoms similar to those they produce". This was called "*the law of similars*".** We now prefer the term "phenomenon of similars" which may be resumed in three propositions.

FIRST PROPOSITION

Every substance, providing that it is **pharmacodynamic**, provokes in the healthy, sensitive individual a set of symptoms which is characteristic of this substance. This was the conclusion of Hahnemann's experiments on healthy subjects.

SECOND PROPOSITION

Every patient presents **a set of morbid symptoms** which is characteristic of his disease.

This declaration might be seen as a statement of the obvious, but Hahnemann adds that "the morbid symptoms should be defined as **the total changes in the way in which the patient feels or behaves as a direct result of his disease**". patient's behavior

What exactly does this mean? For the sake of clarity, let us consider an example, the case of two children who have the measles at the same time.

The two children both have fever, eye and nose irritation, and a characteristic eruption. These symptoms are common to all measles sufferers and the diagnosis of measles is based on them.

But, in fact, as a result of the disease, each child behaves in a different way to when he was healthy; the differences, however, are not necessarily the same in the two cases:

- one may be agitated, the other prostrate;
- one may sweat, the other may not;
- one may be thirsty, the other may not be;
- one may feel hot, the other on the contrary may feel cold and may not be able to warm up in spite of his fever.

For each patient therefore, the homeopathic physician has to consider the **morbid symptoms in their entirety**, that is to say, on the one hand, the **signs which are common** to all children: fever, eye and nose irritation, the characteristic eruption, **as well as**, on the other hand, the **individual signs** proper to each child which are **directly caused by the disease**: agitation or prostration, sweating or dry skin, thirst or lack of thirst, etc.

Disease causes morbid symptoms - common signs - individual signs

This point is fundamental in the understanding and application of the homeopathic method and recurs repeatedly throughout this book.

THIRD PROPOSITION

The recovery of the patient, objectively indicated by the disappearance of all the morbid symptoms, can be achieved by the prescription in small or infinitesimal doses of a substance which provokes symptoms similar to those shown by the patient when administered experimentally to a healthy subject.

It was at this moment, at the beginning of the nineteenth century, that homeopathy was born. It took Hahnemann over ten years of observation and experiments to reach the conclusions summarized in these few lines.

We can see that homeopathy is neither an eccentric idea issued from a crank nor a philosophy, neither a form of mysticism nor a religion. It is quite simply **a therapeutic method, established in the purest tradition of experimental medicine**, and this before the time of Claude Bernard; initially, **the facts viewed objectively** suggested **an idea** and the idea led to **a series of experiments** which in turn **corroborated the idea**.

This therapeutic method consists in giving the patient, in small or infinitesimal doses, the substance which causes similar symptoms to those shown by the patient when administered experimentally to a healthy subject.

This technique may come as a surprise to the reader who is used to the methods of conventional therapeutics. In fact, what usually happens is as follows:

- faced with a patient who is showing troublesome symptoms (fever, pains, spasms, cough, etc.), there is an effort to **inhibit these symptoms chemically** with antipyretics, analgesics, antispasmodics, cough medicines, etc.;
- if it is known that the disease is caused by a microbe, a parasite, etc., an effort will be made **to destroy** the etiologic agent **by chemical means**;
- if the disease engenders a metabolite which is responsible for the symptoms (histamine in allergic phenomena, serotonin in certain types of migraine, etc.,) the treatment will be directed at **chemically combating the excess of the metabolites** or their action with antihistamines, serotonin-inhibiting drugs, etc.;
- if the disease in question is accompanied by an increase in the level of a physiological substance (uric acid, lipids, triglycerides, cholesterol, etc.), again the treatment will **chemically combat** the excess with uricosurics, antilipemics, anticholesterol drugs, etc.;
- and if, on the contrary, the disease is due to a decrease in the normal level of a physiological substance, we would **assume the role** of faltering nature by supplying electrolytes, hormones, synthetic products, etc.

Conventional therapeutics, then, is for the most part expressed by acts of **inhibition, destruction, and substitution**. It is ***coercive or substitutive***.

In homeopathy, on the contrary, **a substance is given to the patient which acts in the same way as the overall reactive mode of the organism, in the same way as the defense mechanisms, in cooperation with them**. It stimulates them to make them more efficient and this is why the substance has to be administered in small if not infinitesimal doses: too strong a dose might unpleasantly aggravate the patient's reactions. ***Homeopathic therapeutics is reactive***.

The two methods may therefore seem *a priori* diametrically opposed. And yet, if we think about it, we can see that conventional therapeutics has often recourse to the phenomenon of similars. Let us consider some examples.

- **Mercury and its salts**, under toxic conditions, provoke phenomena of oliguria and anuria. Conventional therapeutics, until recently, used **mercurial diuretics** to treat oliguria and anuria without of course the treatment being associated with mercury poisoning: hence the parallel between toxicity and therapeutics. Sulfonamide diuretics are more readily used today but the same thing may be said about them.
- **Digitalis** in toxic doses provokes heart disorders with a rapid, irregular rhythm. The most typical indication of digitalin is total arrhythmia due to auricular fibrillation in which, specifically, the ventricular systoles are rapid and irregular: hence, again, the parallel between toxicity and therapeutics.
- **Ergot** is frequently used in conventional therapeutics. Its toxic action, depending on the dose used, includes in sequence:

- vasomotor phenomena accompanied by headaches,
- phenomena of more or less labile arterial hypertension,
- manifestations of arteriopathy accompanied by fixed arterial hypertension and cerebral circulatory insufficiency,
- uterine hemorrhage and serious hemorrhage in the retroperitoneal lumbar fossae,
- and finally, manifestations of arteritis with gangrene in the extremities.

Such is the historical picture of ergotism, St. Anthony's Fire, with its ischemic gangrene provoking burning, hyperalgesic pains.

The indications of ergot in conventional therapeutics are precisely:

- vasomotor headache and migraine,
- arterial hypertension with or without cerebral ischemia,
- uterine hemorrhage.

Again we find the parallel between the toxicological picture and the therapeutic indications. Arteriopathy, however, is a contraindication for the use of ergot in material doses which may provoke a worsening of the morbid phenomena. On the contrary, in homeopathy ergot (*Secale cornutum*) has a very positive indication for arteriopathy because the homeopath has the posology scale of infinitesimal doses at his disposal.

- **Smallpox vaccination** is also a further illustration of the phenomenon of similars because a disease, the vaccine, is inoculated as a preventive measure against smallpox; the disease is clinically manifested through general and cutaneous symptoms similar to those of smallpox, only for a different reason.

And we could continue to enumerate examples, notably in allergology or in immunology where substances capable of provoking pathologic disorders in susceptible subjects are currently used in small doses as therapeutic agents.

This is hardly surprising: the phenomenon of similars is a phenomenon of general biology and it is normal that the practitioner, consciously or unconsciously, should have recourse to it. The only difference between the conventional practitioner and the homeopathic practitioner is that the latter systematically and deliberately seeks to use this phenomenon to maximum advantage.

So the first important point which should be assimilated and constantly borne in mind as far as homeopathic therapeutics is concerned is:

Homeopathy is *a therapeutic method* whose basic principle is based on the *phenomenon of similars* which formulates the parallel between the toxic action of a substance and its therapeutic action.

Logically, for the application of homeopathic therapeutics, this principle implies the knowledge of the action of the various pharmacodynamic substances on a healthy person. This is what is known as **the provings**.

THE PROVINGS

Theoretically, the proving of a substance includes all the symptoms induced by this substance in healthy people. These symptoms come from:

- **intoxication**: it may be acute, chronic, voluntary, accidental, or professional. Given the high doses involved, it mainly produces **organic lesions**.
- **pathogenetic experiments properly speaking**: these are carried out using various non-toxic doses on subjects of different sex and ages, hence of unequal sensitivity. They especially provoke **functional or general symptoms, possibly changes in general behavior**, that is to say, as Hahnemann put it, "**changes in the way of feeling or behaving**".

In practice, however, the provings are supplemented by symptoms originating from a third source:

- **clinical therapeutic observation**: this type of observation has caused the **pathologic symptoms** regularly cured by the substance under study to be included among the provings. But these symptoms also include:
  - firstly, **pathologic symptoms similar to the pathogenetic symptoms produced by a substance and cured by infinitesimal dilutions of this same substance**. In short, they correspond to the "converse" of pathogenetic experimentation, the verification of the phenomenon of similars. These symptoms are of great practical value because they are particularly reliable;
  - secondly, **pathologic symptoms** presented by patients receiving treatment, **unconnected with pathogenetic data, but which have disappeared concomitantly** on the absorption of infinitesimal dilutions of the substance under study which was prescribed for other symptoms.

Let us simply emphasize that this latter provision can certainly be criticized from the methodological point of view. We shall analyze the advantages and disadvantages in *Homeopathic Therapeutics: possibilities in chronic pathology* which is devoted to the treatment of chronic diseases. These drawbacks do not concern the treatment of acute diseases which is the subject of the present volume.

THE SENSITIVE TYPE

Pathogenetic and therapeutic experiments have also enabled homeopaths to identify "**sensitive types**".

These are subjects who, all else being equal, develop more pathogenetic symptoms than the others during the provings in reaction to the same substance.

Observation has shown that these sensitive types may be defined

- according to similar morbid tendencies,
- according to common morphological norms,

- according to comparable traits of character.

This explains why the homeopath may sometimes take the **morphology and general behavior of his patients** into account in his clinical examination as well as the results of conventional semiology. This is especially true for chronic pathology.

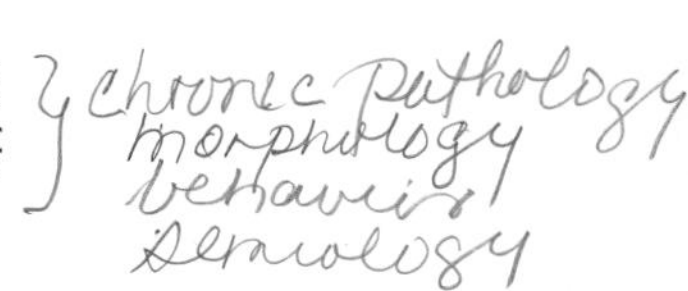

All the symptoms related to the same substance are classified according to the system they affect (digestive, respiratory, cutaneous, etc.) and their totality makes up the proving of the substance. The sum of these provings make up what is known as the **Homeopathic Materia Medica**.

THE HOMEOPATHIC MATERIA MEDICA

This consists of the cataloguing of reactive symptoms, that is to say, "**changes in the way of feeling or behaving**" in healthy people on a local, general, functional, and behavioral levels **under the experimental action** of pharmacodynamic substances.

It is a vast reactive semiology of individuals viewed as **an inseparable whole, a psychosomatic entity, a biological unit**.

In order to practice homeopathic therapeutics, thorough knowledge of the homeopathic materia medica is indispensable to the homeopath.

METHOD OF APPLICATION

With his knowledge of the homeopathic materia medica, the homeopathic physician observes the symptoms of his patient during the illness, i.e. the patient's way of reacting to the complaint. He then prescribes as a remedy dilutions of the substance whose reactive modalities observed during experiments correspond to those of the patient. The remedy thus defined really is "homeopathic" since the basic substance which was used in its preparation is capable of provoking the **same** (homeo) **suffering** (pathos) in a healthy person. And it is essential, if we are to adhere to the rigors of the homeopathic method, to remind ourselves continually that "**homeopathy**" means "**the same suffering**".

Let us now look at a concrete example: two patients consult the doctor for intercostal herpes zoster:

- the first one presents an edematous vesicular eruption and complains of stinging, burning pains which are relieved by applying something cold. The reactive mode of this patient suffering from herpes zoster corresponds exactly to the reactive mode of a healthy person subjected to the toxic action of bee venom. The homeopathic remedy, prepared from a substance likely to cause the same suffering, would be bee venom in an infinitesimal dilution;

- the second patient presents the same eruption and also complains about burning pains. But it is revealed during the casetaking that the pains are worse at night and are relieved by applying something warm. The reactive mode of this patient is therefore totally different from that of the first one, although the nosologic diagnosis is the same. In the homeopathic materia medica this reactive mode corresponds to that of a healthy person subjected to the toxic action of arsenic anhydride (*Arsenicum album*). The homeopathic remedy in this case would be *Arsenicum album* in infinitesimal dilution.

Thus two patients suffering from the same complaint, but who display two different types of behavior and different individual reactive modes during the illness, would have two different types of therapy.

The **homeopathic method consists** then **in superposing two reactive symptomatic pictures** in order to determine which homeopathic remedy or remedies to prescribe:

- **firstly, that of the proving** which is the experimental reactive picture of a healthy person subjected to the action of a pharmacodynamic substance;
- **secondly, the symptomatic picture presented by the patient** which includes not only **the pathognomonic signs of the disease** but also **the specific signs of his personal behavior**. This is the individual reactive picture of the patient during the illness.

THE PATHOGNOMONIC SIGNS OF THE DISEASE

They constitute **conventional semiology** as taught in medical school and include:

- **the physical signs**, that is, the local signs that can be seen, palpated, auscultated, X-rayed, or recorded;
- **the general signs** which stem from the general metabolism of the person: fever, loss of weight, sweating, etc.;
- **the functional signs** which are those felt and expressed by the patient: pain, thirst, asthenia, etc.;
- **the etiologic signs** defined as the **biological norms** which are **common** to all the syndromes constituted by the functional signs; the etiologic signs are revealed by in-depth bacteriological or physiochemical analysis:
    - bacteria, viruses, parasites;
    - abnormally high or low quantities of physiological substances: urea, uric acid, glucose, cholesterol, triglycerides, electrolytes, hormones, etc.;
    - quantitatively abnormal metabolic substances: histamine, serotonin, etc.

These common biological norms are generally considered responsible for the described syndrome even if it is not always known for certain if they are its cause or its consequence.

In any case, the symptomatology taken as a whole makes it possible to establish **the nosologic diagnosis** which **the conventional coercive or substitutive therapeutics** mentioned earlier is based on.

SIGNS SPECIFIC TO THE PATIENT'S BEHAVIOR

These constitute the **homeopathic semiology** which corresponds to the reactive symptoms encountered in the materia medica. Homeopathic semiology includes of course the elements of conventional semiology since these are clinical, objective, and unquestionable, but it will complement them:

- **in the case of physical and general signs**, with ***the modalities***. We use the term "modality" to refer to the qualification of a symptom which shows an aggravation or an improvement due to outside influences, the environment, or the physiological circumstances:
  - heat or cold;
  - rest or movement;
  - time of day: if there is an aggravation or improvement in the morning, after meals, in the evening, at night, etc.;
  - atmospheric conditions: dryness, dampness, sea or mountain climate, etc.;
  - physiological conditions: menstruation, sleep, bowel movements, sweating, etc.
- **in the case of the functional signs**, which depend for their expression on the subjectivity of the patient, ***with the individual's overall sensitivity***; therefore, not only with the modalities of improvement or aggravation of the symptoms but also with an **overview of general behavior**, that is to say, as Hahnemann prescribed, with **"all the changes in the way of feeling or behaving"**(1) **of the patient which are the direct result of his illness**:
  - general behavior: agitation, prostration, sleepiness, aggressiveness, anger, jealousy, seeking of affection or consolation, etc., every phenomenon that we may observe, see, "film", as an objective veterinary doctor might do when examining animals;
  - likes or dislikes for certain foods: thirst or lack of thirst, craving for sweet foods, spices, etc.;
  - sexual behavior;
  - sleep disorders and dreams.

All of these changes should, however, exclude any possible psychiatric or psychoanalytic interpretation.

All these behavioral changes resulting from the disease constitute «nervous symptoms» which some call "psychic symptoms", a term which steers the notion of homeopathic semiology dangerously towards a spurious psychiatric interpretation. We shall return to this subject in *Homeopathic Therapeutics: possibilities in chronic pathology*.

- **in the case of the etiologic signs**, the laboratory results will not be the only data retained for examination. Homeopathic semiology also takes into account the circumstantial

(1) Hahnemann C.S., *Arzneimittellehre*, 1811-1821.

etiology: traumatism, climatic influences, food hygiene, emotional shocks (sorrow, grief, annoyance, fears, etc.); this circumstantial etiology is also known as causality.

Homeopathic semiology will thus define the homeopathic remedy or remedies which will act in the same way as the overall reactive mode of the patient viewed as a biological unit, as an inseparable psychosomatic entity. The homeopathic remedy will therefore optimize the overall individual reactive mode.

The end result of the homeopathic method is an **individualization of therapeutics**.

Homeopathic therapeutics must therefore be considered as **therapeutics of the individual constitution** and **homeopathic medicines** as ***specific regulators of the organism*** compared to conventional medicines which are coercive and substitutive.

Thus the second principal asset of homeopathy which should be kept in mind is ***the method,* which is purely objective and purely clinical**.

This consists in overlaying two reactive symptomatic pictures which can be summarized in two separate reports:

- **the experimental report of the proving,**
- **the complete report on the clinical observation of the patient which brings together conventional semiology and homeopathic semiology.**

Homeopathic semiology **does not replace** conventional semiology which leads to the diagnosis of the disease. **It completes it** with nuances which are specific to each patient and indicate the choice of the homeopathic remedy.

All these notions are summarized in the table on the following page.

It is very important not to lose sight of this table: it rigorously summarizes the method of application of homeopathy and enables the practitioner to avoid methodological blunders. What is more, it highlights three important points:

1. **It shows that homeopathy is not a form of therapeutics only based on symptoms** as some uninformed doctors have reproached it for being. It rejects neither nosologic diagnosis nor etiology. As for the latter, homeopathic semiology pays attention to elements which are not retained in conventional semiology.
2. **It shows that there is no equation, that there are no automatic links**, between the diagnosis of the disease and its treatment. In fact, the individual reactive mode of the patient should always intervene between the nosologic diagnosis and the choice of the homeopathic remedy. This explains why in this therapeutics handbook the reader will find several possible homeopathic remedies for the same complaint, for the same pathologic background. These remedies, under experimental conditions, have as their chosen pathogenetic targets the organs, functions, and tissues which are affected by the disease in question, **accompanied, as the case may be, by similar anatomicopathological lesions**. This does not of course mean that the doctor should prescribe them all. Each of these possible medicines affects pathogenetic targets with its own modalities. It is the responsibility of the homeopathic physician to prescribe the remedy or remedies whose experimental modalities correspond best to the individual reactive modalities of the patient.

3. **It specifies the indications and the limits of homeopathic therapeutics**: since the homeopathic remedy is a specific stimulant of the organism, homeopathic therapeutics should be applied each time the person's defense system is potentially able to confront the morbid aggression. This involves approximately 70 to 80% of the sum total of patients. Conventional therapeutics, which is coercive or substitutive, should only be used in the 20 to 30% of remaining cases, in which affected organisms are suffering physiological distress and the person's defense system can no longer cope. Its effectiveness is remarkable in these serious cases but as its use is not devoid of toxic side effects it should be reserved exclusively for them.

Certainly, there is no sharp dividing line between these two groups of patients: there is a fringe group of cases for which one is allowed and, indeed, has the duty, to combine the two forms of therapeutics since they do not act at the same level.

When justified by clinical necessity, there is nothing incompatible nor heretical in combining homeopathic therapeutics and conventional therapeutics.

The homeopathic physician is first and foremost a physician. He is skilled in using two therapeutic tools. It is his duty to use them in the best possible way in the best interests of his patient.

PATHOGENETIC REPORT

TOXICOLOGY + **CLINICAL AND PATHOGENETIC EXPERIMENTATION**

physical symptoms of lesion

general and functional symptoms

"changes in the manner of feeling or behaving"

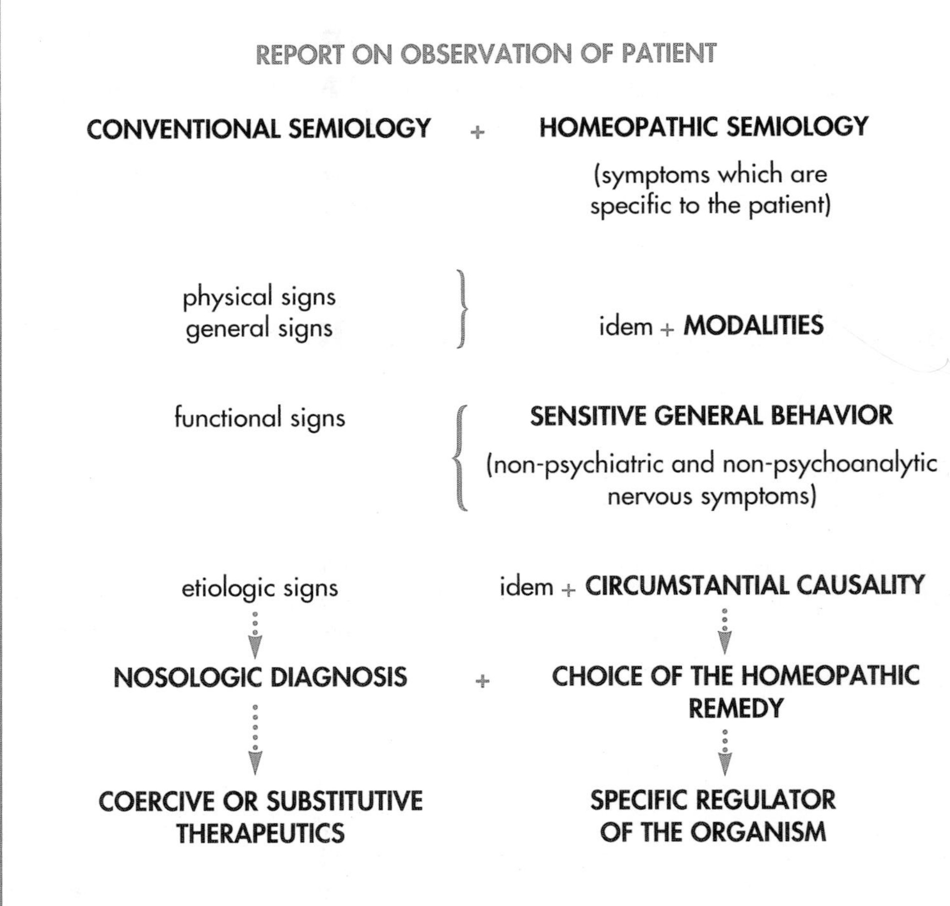

CHAPTER II

PRACTICAL APPLICATIONS

Now that the general principles and basic definitions have been explained, it is necessary to respect these clearly defined rules in daily medical practice so that homeopathic principles can be applied rigorously. To do this, the homeopathic practitioner should always bear in mind that:

A. HOMEOPATHY IS A THERAPEUTIC METHOD BASED ON THE PHENOMENON OF SIMILARS.

It consists in giving the patient, as a medicine, the substance which is likely to produce **similar** (homeo) **suffering** (pathos) in a healthy and/or sensitive individual.

B. THE METHOD HAS THREE ORIGINAL FEATURES.

FIRST ORIGINAL FEATURE

This is to be acquainted with the symptoms provoked under experimental conditions in healthy and sensitive subjects by the different pharmacodynamic substances, that is to **know the provings** which, taken as a whole, constitute the **homeopathic materia medica**.

SECOND ORIGINAL FEATURE

This is to understand in the expression "similar suffering", "**the sum of changes in the way of feeling or behaving of the patient which are a direct result of his disease**", that is, not only the pathognomonic signs of the diseases to treat - those which correspond to conventional semiology - but also the individual reactive symptoms which are specific to each patient as a direct result of his disease - **those which constitute homeopathic semiology**.

THIRD ORIGINAL FEATURE

With this definition of the homeopathic remedy, which acts in the same way as the overall reactive mode of the patient viewed as a biological unit and an inseparable psychosomatic entity, it is essential to resort to **infinitesimal doses**.

Hence, in practice, the homeopathic practitioner confronted with a patient should never ask himself, "What are the homeopathic remedies to prescribe for such a nosologic complaint?", but "What are the substances which, when administered to a healthy person, provoke similar symptoms to those of the patient?"

We are now going to take a closer look at each of these three original features of the homeopathic method.

CHAPTER III

FIRST ORIGINAL FEATURE: THE PROVINGS

In recent decades, some authors have successively managed to classify the accumulation of symptoms which could be found in old books on homeopathic materia medica. They have been able to show that in fact each pharmacodynamic substance, whether it belongs to the botanical, biological, or mineral kingdoms, presents, depending on its toxicity, an affinity for a particular organ, function, or tissue. They have been able to state that these substances in some way have specific targets.

In the first instance, the student should get acquainted with **the pathogenetic targets**.

He will then notice very quickly that the same organ, function, or tissue may be affected by several different substances in toxic or pharmaceutical doses.

But each of these substances acts upon the targets in question in its own specific way, that is according to the modalities which are characteristic of the substance tested.

Secondly, he must also learn what the **characteristic modalities** are.

From that moment, with his knowledge on the one hand of the reciprocal affinities of certain organs or physiological functions and certain pharmacodynamic substances and, on the other hand, of the characteristic modalities of their action, the student will be able to see the emergence of the third stage of homeopathic practice **which allows the logical deduction of the therapeutic possibilities** of the substance tested according to the phenomenon of similars.

As far as the prescription is concerned, the dosage will be based upon the general principles described further on.

As an example we are going to study, following this schema, the eight main remedies for acute fever. Four of the remedies correspond especially to febrile conditions with a sudden onset: *Aconitum*, *Belladonna*, *Apis*, and *Arsenicum album*. Four remedies correspond to febrile conditions with a more progressive onset: *Bryonia*, *Rhus toxicodendron*, *Gelsemium*, and *Ferrum phosphoricum*.

This will enable the reader to acquire a working method that he can apply - by personally preparing similar summaries - to the other remedies used in the homeopathic treatment of acute diseases presented in the second part of this book

REMEDIES FOR ACUTE PYREXIA WITH A SUDDEN ONSET

ACONITUM NAPELLUS

This plant belongs to the Ranunculaceae family; its principal alkaloid, aconitine, is particularly toxic.

PATHOGENETIC ACTION (THE TARGETS)

- **circulatory sphere**: congestive irritability with:
  - acceleration and fullness of the pulse;
  - arterial hypertension with a red and bloated face and active congestion of the different viscera (digestive ++);
  - possible hemorrhages of bright, red, warm blood.
- **nervous sphere**: excitation caused by bulbar and spinal congestion and irritation of sensory nerves, therefore:
  - **general excitation with anxiety,** vertigo, fear in general, and, in acute states, fear of death because of the severe and intense general signs felt by the subject during experimentation;
  - **neuralgic phenomena** with numbness, tingling sensation, then anesthesia. Elective localization in the trigeminal nerve.

MODALITIES AND CHARACTERISTIC SIGNS

- **sudden hyperthermia which often starts with shivering**;
- **red, dry skin, without perspiration**;
- **intense thirst for large quantities of cold water**;
- **intense agitation with anxiety and fear of death,** because of the intensity of the clinical phenomena.

AGGRAVATION

- with keen and/or sudden cold;
- at about midnight.

IMPROVEMENT

- when perspiration starts in acute conditions. This remedy is then no longer indicated; *Belladonna* is indicated if there is no drop in temperature.

SENSATIONS

- of acute, unbearable pains;
- of numbness, of tingling.

LIKES AND DISLIKES

- in acute conditions, unquenchable thirst for cold water since everything but water tastes bitter.

MAIN CLINICAL INDICATIONS

Aconitum napellus is the remedy to be prescribed in the following cases:
- first stage of defense mechanisms, before any clinical localization which could evoke a nosologic diagnosis;
- congestive or hypertensive rashes;
- neuralgia triggered by cold.

1. ACUTE FEBRILE CONDITION

Whatever the diagnosis and the etiology (microbial or viral):
- onset of rhinopharyngitis, tonsillitis;
- onset of laryngitis or bronchitis (with croupy cough +++);
- acute diarrhea, etc.

Depending on similarity and the seriousness of the case, prescribe a dilution between 5C and 30C, five pellets every half-hour or every hour, until the symptoms disappear or sweating begins.

2. PAROXYSTIC CARDIOVASCULAR CONDITION

Hypertensive attack:
- paroxysmal headache with or without sluggishness;
- tachycardia with irritability;
- precordial pain.

Historically, *Aconitum* was called "the homeopathic lancet". Prescribe five pellets every two to six hours in 9 or 15C depending on intensity and similarity.

3. NEURALGIA TRIGGERED BY COLD

Prescribe in 15 or 30C every 2 to 6 hours.

4. AMENORRHEA AFTER A SUDDEN CHILL

Prescribe four doses with a "scaled dosage": one dose in 9C on the first day, one dose in 12C on the second day, one dose in 15C on the third day, and one dose in 30C on the fourth day.

BELLADONNA

Atropa belladonna is a plant of the Solanaceae family. It contains two principal alkaloids which are very toxic, atropine and hyoscyamine; they have **a powerful parasympatholytic action which dominates and explains the entire proving.**

PATHOGENETIC ACTION

- **on the mucous membranes**: secretions diminish, and so the mucous membranes are dry.
- **on the vascular system**: belladonna in toxic doses causes intense phenomena of congestion:
  - **local**: it produces the clinical picture of local inflammation: rubor, tumor, dolor, calor;

- **cephalic**: red face, cerebral hyperemia;
- **general**: scarlatiniform rash, tachycardia with irritability, fever which may induce convulsions, sweating, and dejection and agitation alternately.

- **on the nervous system**:
  - **the central system**: general sensory hyperesthesia;
  - **the sympathetic system**: tachycardia ++, mydriasis, spasms of the smooth or striated muscular fibers (sphincters, hollow organs, musculotendinous apparatus).

Belladonna corresponds to the second stage of the general defense reactions: **inflammation.**

MODALITIES AND CHARACTERISTIC SYMPTOMS

AGGRAVATION

- with light;
- with noise;
- with touch (direct contact or abrupt movements);
- with cold air.

The patient's general sensory hyperesthesia accounts for all these reactive modalities.

IMPROVEMENT

- with rest;
- in a half-sitting position.

SENSATIONS

- pulsating, throbbing pains, which are characteristic of congestion;
- dryness of the mucous membranes;
- cramp-like, spasmodic pains **which begin and end suddenly.**

LIKES AND DISLIKES

The patient may experience different types of thirst during febrile conditions. The thirst is therefore never characteristic, as with *Aconitum* for example. But depending on its characteristics, it might be an indication of the remedy to be administered afterwards, which will supplement the action of *Belladonna*:

- *Bryonia* if there is intense thirst for large quantities of cold water;
- *Arsenicum album* if there is thirst for small but frequent quantities;
- *Gelsemium* or *Apis*: the patient is not thirsty.

We will return later in the book to the necessity of almost always using several remedies alternately with the same patient. This may be easily explained and understood from a physiopathologic point of view.

PRINCIPAL CLINICAL INDICATIONS

1. ALL TYPES OF FEVER WITH A SUDDEN AND VIOLENT ONSET

Homeopathic treatment with *Belladonna* should be envisaged for any person - adult, child, or baby - who goes to bed in good health but wakes up a few hours later with an acute febrile condition.

In practice this picture corresponds to the invasion phase in almost all infectious diseases.

2. INTENSE LOCAL OR GENERAL VASCULAR CONGESTION

local:
- onset of inflammation, of abscess;
- cephalic congestion because of sunstroke, hot flushes, or hypertensive attacks.

general:
- fluctuant, relapsing fever, with a red face, profuse sweating, alternate dejection and agitation (delirium);
- scarlatinifom rash.

This may occur during rhinopharyngitis, tonsillitis (with dryness and spasms in the throat), eruptive diseases during the phase of invasion or eruption: scarlet fever, measles, etc.

3. DRYNESS OF MUCOUS MEMBRANES

- rhinopharyngitis, tonsillitis, onset of tracheitis.

4. SPASMODIC PHENOMENA

- musculotendinous jolts,
- hiccups,
- spasms of hollow organs,
- febrile convulsions.

DOSAGE

In accordance with the general rules (see p. 67):
- **with restricted or local symptoms**: prescribe five pellets in 5C every 1 to 4 hours, depending on the severity of the case;
- **with more extensive symptoms** (associated general signs, nervous spasms), prescribe in 9C every 1 to 4 hours;
- **to prevent febrile convulsions** in children who are prone to them, prescribe in 15 or 30C every hour.

In every case, increase the interval between doses according to improvement.

APIS MELLIFICA

The mother tincture (MT) is prepared by macerating the whole bee in alcohol. It has a very complex composition and contains histamine, dopamine, and noradrenaline which play a role in edema and acute inflammatory reactions.

PATHOGENETIC ACTION

The experimental toxic action of *Apis mellifica* resembles the sting of a bee which can cause the following lesions depending on how sensitive the person is:
- **on the skin**: stinging, burning, red-pink edema with a sudden onset;
- **on the mucous membranes**: edema which is clinically spectacular (eyelids, genital area) or dramatic (edema of the glottis);
- **on the serous membranes**: exudative reaction which may cause more or less abundant effusion: pleurisy, pericarditis, meningitis, etc.;
- **on the urogenital tract**: the renal parenchyma is affected in the case of edematous nephritis; the ovaries (mainly the right one) are affected.

CHARACTERISTIC MODALITIES

- the symptoms appear **very suddenly**;

- **red-pink edema with stinging, burning pain**;
- **improvement with cold** and aggravation with warmth;
- in febrile conditions:
  - **absence of thirst,**
  - **dry, warm skin and episodes of sweating, alternately.**

PRINCIPAL CLINICAL INDICATIONS

1. *CUTANEOUS*

- local edematous complaints: insect bites, sunburn, furuncle or whitlow at their onset;
- more general complaints: urticaria, erysipelas.

Common factors: edema and pruritus improved with cold.

2. *MUCOUS MEMBRANES*

- conjunctivitis, keratitis;
- tonsillitis with edema of the uvula or of the glottis (in this case, the patient does not feel thirsty but the local pain is improved with cold drinks);
- vaginitis, balanitis.

Common factors: edema improved with cold; fever but absence of thirst.

3. *SEROUS MEMBRANES*

- hydrarthrosis with a pinkish red edema of the joint;
- pleurisy, pericarditis with fever but no thirst;
- mumps meningitis: very clear indication because of violent headache, state of stupor and even unconsciousness, red, congested face; the head is restless and rolls from side to side on the pillow;
- it is useful to add *Apis* to conventional therapy for all types of meningeal edema if the reactive mode is similar to the pathogenetic process.

4. *UROGENITAL TRACT*

- acute nephritis with oliguria, albuminuria, edema with no thirst;
- oophoritis, mainly on the right side (*Bryonia*).

DOSAGE

All the dilutions are active but it is better to use high dilutions since some individuals are allergic to bee venom. Allergologists have reported that some patients are sensitive to dilutions of 10^{-14}, that is to say 7C; therefore dilutions of less than 9C are never used in practice. Prescribe dilutions of 9 or 15C, in doses of five pellets every 10 to 30 minutes in acute cases, increasing the intervals with improvement; in subacute or chronic cases, five pellets two to four times a day.

The remedy acts fast but its effect is only temporary.

Remember that *Apis* has an anti-inflammatory action similar to the action of antihistamines, phenylbutazone, and corticoids when tested on animals.

ARSENICUM ALBUM

This is arsenic anhydride, As_2O_3, a particularly violent poison; the acute homeopathic indications were revealed by the pathogenetic symptoms studied in toxicology.

PATHOGENETIC ACTION

Arsenic anhydride has a very extensive and profound pharmacologic action which can affect practically all the organs and all the physiological functions. It causes a febrile reaction, as well as:

- **ulcerous, necrotizing type of irritation in the mucous membranes**:
  - **digestive**: vomiting, choleriform and bloody diarrhea;
  - **respiratory**: mainly nasopharynx and bronchi;
  - **urogenital**: cystitis, hematuria, vaginitis, etc.;
- **the noble parenchyma is affected**:
  - **kidneys**: oliguria, albuminuria, hematuria, nephritis with cylindruria;
  - **liver**: cellular degeneration or cytolysis;
  - **suprarenal**: hypotension, asthenia;
- **the nervous system is also affected**:
  - **convulsions and coma** in acute intoxication;
  - **progressive paralysis** with cramps in prolonged subacute intoxication.

MODALITIES AND CHARACTERISTIC SIGNS

- **burning pain** as with hot embers, **relieved by heat**;
- **acrid, burning, excoriating, and putrid secretions;**
- **all the phenomena are aggravated at night between one and three in the morning;**
- **weakness, pallor, sensitivity to cold, prostration, and anxious agitation alternately with fear of death because of the severe toxic syndrome;**
- **intense thirst** for "small but frequent quantities of water".

AGGRAVATION

- **with cold**, cold food and chilled drinks;
- **at night between one and three in the morning.**

IMPROVEMENT

- **with heat** in any form: applying something warm, warmth from a source of heat, warm drinks or food;
- with changes in position or place (agitation).

SENSATIONS

- **of intense burning**, "as with hot embers";
- **of extreme weakness.**

EXCRETIONS AND SECRETIONS

- **moderate, fluid, burning, foul**, with a cadaverous odor.

LIKES AND DISLIKES

- **longing for cold water**.

PRINCIPAL CLINICAL INDICATIONS

The main feature is a severely affected general condition with extreme weakness and intensely acute burning pains:

- **acute gastroenteritis**, food poisoning due to **rotten meat or canned food**, shellfish;
- acute cystitis (*Cantharis, Mercurius corrosivus)*; nephritis;
- metritis, acute or subacute vaginitis;
- **nocturnal attack of asthma** (if the modalities of the remedy are present);
- burning, **acute, cutaneous manifestations**, with a severely affected overall condition: furuncle, anthrax, erysipelas, herpes zoster, septic stings, etc. (*Pyrogenium, Tarentula cubensis, Lachesis)*;
- severe, typhus-like, septic infectious conditions of whatever origin if accompanied by weakness, anxious agitation, sensitivity to cold, burning pains improved by heat.

DOSAGE

Depending on the degree of similarity, prescribe in 5, 9, or 15 C, five pellets once or several times a day depending on the severity of the case. Conventional therapy will of course also be prescribed if necessary, for particularly severe cases where the patient's defenses are too weak to fight the morbid effects of the disease.

REMEDIES FOR ACUTE PYREXIA WITH A PROGRESSIVE ONSET

BRYONIA ALBA

This is white bryony, a plant of the Cucurbitaceae family.

PATHOGENETIC ACTION

Bryony causes essentially three experimental phenomena:

- **dryness of the mucous membranes**: mainly the respiratory and digestive membranes. It dries up secretions and causes a characteristic dryness which is why the subjects felt so **thirsty** in all the experiments. The **underlying cellular tissue** is sometimes concomitantly inflamed, as in the first phase of phlegmonous reactions;
- **inflammation and exudation of the serous membranes** (pleura, pericardium, peritoneum, synovial membranes...) which may also affect the adjoining organs; the subjects under experiment **try to keep still** to reduce the pain;

- **adynamic febrile syndrome**: attempt to remain immobile, intense thirst, dejection, sweating.

MODALITIES AND CHARACTERISTIC SIGNS

AGGRAVATION

- **with movement**,
- with the slightest touch,
- **with heat in any form**, except for local pain which is relieved by applying heat,
- in the evening at about nine.

IMPROVEMENT

- **with rest**,
- **with strong pressure** or lying on the painful side,
- with cold,
- with sweating.

SENSATIONS

- **of acute, stinging, nagging pain,** worsened by the slightest movement or the slightest touch, and improved with wide and continuous pressure, heat, and rest.

LIKES

- **intense thirst for large quantities of cold water** during febrile episodes.

LATERAL DOMINANCE

- prevailing right-hand side.

PRINCIPAL CLINICAL INDICATIONS

1. *FEVER*

Bryonia is indicated in all febrile conditions, whether continuous or remittent, with a rather progressive onset, during which the patient is dejected, tired, and irritable, and **tries to remain still**. Whatever the cause, this remedy is indicated when the patient's clinical reactive mode has the following characteristics corresponding to the experimental pathogenetic modalities:

- **extreme dryness of all the mucous membranes with intense thirst**;
- **increased pain with the slightest movement**: the patient tries to remain immobile; **headache**, which is mainly frontal, is aggravated by coughing or by the slightest movement of the eyeballs;
- oily, profuse, **sour sweat which brings relief;**
- **sometimes delirium** when the fever is high.

Prescribe in 9, or 15C according to similarity, five pellets two to four times a day.

2. *ACUTE ARTHRITIS*

with the characteristic reactive modalities:

- **warm, red, swollen joints**; the pain is relieved by applying something warm, which distinguishes *Bryonia* from *Apis mellifica*.

In practice, however, it is better to alternate these two remedies if the patient does not show a characteristic modality of improvement or aggravation with cold or warmth. Indeed, they have **the same experimental action on the articular serous membranes, the same anatomicopathological affinity**.

These medicines often have a spectacular anti-inflammatory action.

3. *PLEURISY, SEROFIBRINOUS PLEURISY AT THE ONSET, PLEUROPNEUMONIA*

When the following signs are present:

- a painful stitch aggravated by movement or respiration;
- improvement with pressure or with lying on the painful side;
- intense thirst.

In these complaints, the action of *Bryonia* is conveniently complemented by *Sulphur iodatum 9C*, five pellets a day.

4. TRACHEITIS OR BRONCHITIS

When the patient shows:
- a dry, painful cough, worsened by the slightest movement;
- aggravated when entering a warm room;
- with retrosternal or thoracic pain relieved by compressing the thorax with both hands to stop it from moving (*Drosera*).

5. ABDOMINAL COMPLAINTS

- febrile gastric disorders with nausea, vomiting, or diarrhea triggered by the slightest movement; very bitter taste in the mouth and intense thirst;
- **in acute cholecystitis** and typhoid *Bryonia* can be very helpful in association with conventional therapy.

6. ACUTE MASTITIS

- with heavy breasts that are painful with the slightest movement.

DOSAGE

For all these indications, follow the general rules for dosage which are explained later in the book (see p. 67):
- **in the case of local similarity**, use **low dilutions** (5C) with frequently repeated doses depending on the severity of the case;
- **in the case of similarity with general signs or characteristic modalities**, use **medium dilutions** (9C);
- **in the case of extended similarity, including symptoms of nervous behavior**, use **high dilutions** (15 or 30C).

RHUS TOXICODENDRON

This is poison sumac, a shrub of the Anacardiaceae family; the plant contains a particularly caustic latex.

PATHOGENETIC ACTION

Toxicology and experimentation have shown an elective action on:
- **the skin**, where it causes edema and vesicular eruption;

- **the mucous membranes**, which it irritates;
- **the periarticular fibrous and connective tissue** (tendons, ligaments, aponeurosis), where it causes **painful stiffness improved by movement**;
- **the nervous system**, which it depresses; this depression is manifested in **febrile conditions** by an **adynamic syndrome** with both prostration and agitation; this apparent antinomy can be explained by the reactive modalities of the remedy.

MODALITIES AND CHARACTERISTIC SIGNS

IMPROVEMENT

- **with slow movement, with a change in position**, for pruritus in cutaneous lesions, articular pain, or phenomena accompanying fever;
- **with heat and with applying something warm**;
- with warm, dry weather.

AGGRAVATION

- **with humidity**, damp cold, **wet contact**;
- with rest and immobility;
- **with starting to move and excessive tiredness**.

These aggravating factors are so characteristic that they may be sufficient for the choice of the remedy; they may in themselves be the prime reason for prescribing it.

CAUSALITIES

- **chill** caused by humidity or **after getting soaked**: bath, rain;
- chill caused by sweating after exertion;
- muscular overexertion.

SENSATIONS

- **of myalgia, injury, stiffness, numbness**;
- of cold water thrown on the body or on certain parts of the body.

LIKES

- **cold drinks**: cold water, cold milk which may cause shivering after ingestion.

CUTANEOUS SYMPTOMS

- **eruption of small vesicles which contain a transparent, citrine liquid**. The vesicles, about one millimeter in diameter, sit on a base which is burning, pruritic, and erythematous; they are relieved by **applying something warm, by showers or baths**, but not by scratching;
- **"leopard skin" eruptions**: erythematous aspect interspersed with healthy skin.

MUCOUS SYMPTOMS

- **hoarseness when starting to speak** or to sing, which then improves;
- during febrile episodes, **dryness of the mouth, pharynx, and tongue** which is covered with a brown or whitish coating leaving a **red triangle at the tip**;
- intense thirst for cold water or milk;
- diarrhea with scanty, glairy, blood-streaked, extremely nauseous stools, with a burning sensation in the rectum; sensitivity of the caecum and of the right iliac fossa.

PERIARTICULAR SYMPTOMS

The serous membranes are not affected by *Rhus toxicodendron*, but they are by *Bryonia*.

- **sensation of painful articular stiffness, relieved by movement**. The pain is still there or gets worse at the start of the movement, but then decreases, as if relieved by the patient loosening up, and returns with tiredness. **Improvement with warmth and aggravation with humidity**. (These sensations may appear during a rheumatismal episode or after violent exercise. In the latter case, *Arnica* may also be prescribed. But with *Arnica*, the sensations of injury and myalgia are **muscular** and not articular, and movement does not relieve the pain);
- **sciatica with tearing pain**, tugging all along the nerve; **rest makes it worse and movement relieves it**. *Rhus toxicodendron* is indicated for example for lumbar pain or for lumbar sciatica following exposure to the rain or after a chill due to sweating from exertion.

ADYNAMIC FEBRILE SYNDROME

- **state of stupor, prostration, with agitation**, because of the pain endured in the area where the body is in contact with the bed; **the patient tries to move and constantly changes position or place to relieve the pain**;
- **he starts shivering at the slightest movement or when he is even only slightly uncovered**; there is an accompanying dry cough;
- general sweating everywhere except on the face;
- dry tongue with a brown or whitish coat except on the tip; **intense thirst for cold water** or for cold milk which provokes coughing and shivering;
- **herpes around the mouth**.

●●●●●●●●●●●●●●●

Rhus toxicodendron is one of the "trio of restless remedies" described by Nash(2) along with *Aconitum napellus* and *Arsenicum album*:
- the *Aconitum* patient is restless because he is sthenic and vigorous but at the same time worried about his intense general symptoms which make him fear a fatal disease;
- the *Arsenicum* patient is restless mainly during the night and then goes through phases of extreme general weakness, which also make him fear a fatal disease;
- the *Rhus toxicodendron* patient is restless because his pain is relieved by movement.

MAIN CLINICAL INDICATIONS

1. *CUTANEOUS OR MUCOUS COMPLAINTS*

- all types of edematous and/or vesicular dermatosis with the aspect and modalities of the remedy: **eczema, herpes, herpes zoster**, erysipelas, acne rosacea;
- **phlyctenular conjunctivitis, phlyctenular keratitis.**

Prescribe in 9C two to four times a day depending on the severity of the symptoms.

2. *ARTICULAR COMPLAINTS*

- muscular or tendinous **rheumatism**;
- **sprain, luxation** (*Ruta graveolens*);
- tendency towards muscular fatigue; muscular overexertion (the overstrained heart of an athlete);

(2) Nash E.B., *Leaders in Homeopathic Therapeutics*, Boericke & Tafel, Philadelphia - 1898.

- **rheumatism caused and/or aggravated by humidity**.

Same dosage. The 15C dilution is sometimes more effective for rheumatic indications.

ADYNAMIC FEBRILE CONDITION

- **influenza, influenzal conditions**, any microbial or viral complaint for which the clinical reactive modes correspond to the pathogenetic symptoms of the remedy.

Prescribe in 9C, five pellets every two hours approximately.

GELSEMIUM SEMPERVIRENS

This is **yellow jasmine**, a creeping shrub of the Loganiaceae family. This plant is extremely poisonous, especially the roots and bark.

PATHOGENETIC ACTION

Intoxication causes:

- **an adynamic febrile syndrome** accompanied by sphincteral incontinence and obnubilation;
- **paralysis of the motor nerves**, because of histologic lesion of the anterior horns of the spinal cord; this is followed by
- **paralysis of the respiratory muscles;** the patient then dies of cardiac arrest.

The provings revealed:

- **a specific action on the cerebrospinal nervous system** accompanied by:
  - **excitation in the first phase**: **tremor**, cramps, problems of coordination;
  - **paresis in the second phase because of passive congestion** of the brain and the spinal cord: general prostration and heaviness in all the limbs;
- **an action on the circulatory system**: a slowing down of the cardiac rhythm and hypotension;
- **an action on the respiratory and digestive mucous membranes**: it causes a more or less pronounced catarrhal inflammation.

MODALITIES AND CHARACTERISTIC SIGNS

SENSATIONS

- **of weariness, drowsiness, and general numbness**, accompanied by extreme weakness;
- **of myalgia** all over the body and the limbs, which feel extremely heavy;
- **of headache with a crimson, congested face**, and an impression that the head is full and the extremities cold;
- **of diplopia**;
- that the heart is about to stop beating if the subject does not move.

CAUSALITIES

- **depressing emotions**; *Coffea*, however, is indicated for the after-effects of joyful emotions or good news; the nervous system in the latter cases is in the same highly excitable condition as that caused by caffeine in toxic doses;
- **nervous apprehension**, anxiety due to anticipation;
- **chill** after having been too hot; *Aconitum* and *Belladonna* are more often indicated in complaints with a sudden onset, after a cold wave during hard winters for example; *Gelsemium* is indicated for less violent chills with a more progressive onset.

AGGRAVATION

- **with heat**, with warm weather;
- **with emotions, bad news.**

IMPROVEMENT

- **with profuse urination**;
- **with sweating**;
- with movement or sudden jolts (mainly when the cardiac rhythm has slowed down).

LIKES AND DISLIKES

- **the patient does not feel thirsty in acute febrile conditions.**

MAIN CLINICAL INDICATIONS

Depending on the toxicological data, *Gelsemium* is more especially indicated in the following cases:

- **all adynamic infectious conditions**, in particular adynamic encephalitic influenza;
- **localized motor paralysis**.

According to the pathogenetic data, it is particularly indicated for:

- **nervous apprehension** and its consequences;
- **migraine or congestive headaches**.

1. INFLUENZA IN ITS ADYNAMIC FORM

- **prostrate and trembling subject**: tremor is sometimes spectacular and the patient is so prostrate that any movement tires him out;
- **crimson-red face**, with stupor, heavy eyelids, and cold extremities;
- **myalgia** and heaviness of the limbs;
- **shivering** up and down the spine;
- **intense headache** spreading to the neck and the shoulders;
- **absence of thirst**.

Prescribe five pellets in 9C every two hours approximately.

2. NERVOUS APPREHENSION

- before examinations or social obligations;
- before dental or surgical care.

Gelsemium is indicated when there is **sluggishness, forgetfulness**, the impression that the legs are giving way, and a **tendency towards diarrhea** as well as nervous apprehension.

Prescribe a dose of *Gelsemium 30C* on the preceding evening and a second dose one or two hours before the ordeal. In cases of nervous anticipation, prescribe a weekly dose of *Gelsemium 30C* for 3 or 4 weeks before the ordeal, with possibly also five pellets of *Ignatia 9C* every day, then the doses in 30C, as indicated previously, the day before and on the day of the ordeal.

HEADACHES AND MIGRAINES

When they are:

- **congestive**, with **visual disorders (diplopia)** and heavy eyelids before the onset of the headache;

- **with painful eyeballs** which feel damaged (*Eupatorium perfoliatum* is used when the eyeballs are painful with pressure);
- mainly occipital, spreading to the muscles of the neck and the shoulders;
- **relieved** when the head is upright or by **urinating profusely**.

Prescribe five pellets in 9C, two to four times a day, according to how serious the symptoms are.

FERRUM PHOSPHORICUM

This is ferrosoferric phosphate.

PATHOGENETIC ACTION

Experimentation has revealed possible hemorrhagic phenomena which can be related to the presence of phosphorous ions, and pronounced asthenia accompanied by vasomotor phenomena which can be explained by the presence of ferric ions.

Ferrum phosphoricum is indicated for **inflammatory conditions** accompanied by **fairly moderate fever**, with a **tendency to congestion or localized hemorrhage**. It corresponds to the first stage of inflammation, like *Aconitum* or *Belladonna*, but the clinical reactions are less intense, less sudden, and more discreet, because the patient is far less sthenic than the patients for whom these two remedies are indicated.

Ferrum phosphoricum is indicated most of the time for pale, anemic, **tired children or adolescents** with a tendency towards bleeding (epistaxis). The adynamia of the febrile condition of *Ferrum phosphoricum* can be explained by the weakness of the patient's reactions, whereas in the case of *Gelsemium*, *Bryonia*, or *Rhus toxicodendron* it can be explained by the seriousness of the disease.

MODALITIES AND CHARACTERISTIC SIGNS

- **moderate temperature**, less than 39°C;
- **fast but supple and soft pulse**;
- the face is **alternately red and pale**; the skin is generally moist;
- **the patient has a tendency towards hemorrhaging** and particularly to **epistaxis**; there are localized phenomena of congestion, mainly in the ears (congestive otitis) or in the air passages (tracheitis or bronchitis cough);

- **spasmodic, very painful, dry cough**, with stinging, burning pain in the chest; aggravation with cold air or in a lying position; expectoration is yellow and sometimes streaked with blood;
- pain in the right shoulder and the right arm.

MAIN CLINICAL INDICATIONS

- **febrile or inflammatory complaints** in the first stage; eruptive diseases during the phases of incubation or invasion;
- **congestive acute otitis** (with *Capsicum* and *Oscillococcinum*®);
- **tracheitis and bronchitis** (alternating with *Bryonia*).

In all these acute indications, prescribe *Ferrum phosphoricum 9C*, five pellets one to four times a day depending on the severity of the symptoms.

For children with a tendency towards epistaxis or repetitive congestive otitis, prescribe a dose in 9C one to three times a week.

● ● ● ● ● ● ● ● ● ● ● ● ● ● ● ●

At the end of the schematic study of these eight remedies for acute fever, the reader will have noticed that each medicine is indicated for very different complaints.

This may seem puzzling at first. In the course of his conventional medical studies, the practitioner is used to studying therapeutics according to the nosologic diagnosis or to the etiology of the disease. Conversely, each conventional remedy usually corresponds to a disease, to a well-defined group of diseases, or to a specific physiological process: antibiotic, anti-inflammatory, antihistamine, etc.

As Dr. Denis Demarque emphasized(3), it is important to understand that, in keeping with the definition of homeopathy and in keeping with the method of application described in the previous pages, the homeopathic remedy is almost never specific to a nosologically-defined complaint, a microbe, bacterium, virus, or allergen.

It is essential to remember that ***the homeopathic remedy can only be specific to three conditions***:

- either **a stage in the inflammatory process or lesion**;
- or **a localization of inflammation or lesion**: some remedies have a specific pharmacologic affinity for a particular organ or tissue;
- or **a global reactive mode**, that is to say **a constitution**.

(3) Dr. Denis Demarque, *Homéopathie, Médecine de l'expérience* 2ème édition, Maisonneuve, 1982.

The special modalities of each homeopathic remedy, at each of these three levels, define in fact as many **particular clinical forms**, and different precise reactive modes, as we need to **adapt and individualize our homeopathic prescription**.

CHAPTER IV

SECOND ORIGINAL FEATURE: "SIMILAR SUFFERING" = CONVENTIONAL SEMIOLOGY + HOMEOPATHIC SEMIOLOGY

HOW CAN THIS EQUATION BE SOLVED PRACTICALLY?

······➤ BY APPROPRIATE CASETAKING AND EXAMINATION.

In chapter I it was emphasized that homeopathic semiology is not a substitute for conventional semiology which leads to a nosologic diagnosis, but supplements it with particular nuances which are specific to the patient and indicate the choice of the homeopathic remedy.

In practice, therefore, the homeopathic practitioner should carry out his clinical examination just like the conventional practitioner and he should also conduct a special in-depth inquiry which will allow him to identify exactly the particular, individual nuances **specific to the behavior of the patient during his illness**.

This particular technique of casetaking and examination may be summed up by Hering's diagram in the form of a St. Andrew's cross in which each quadrant refers to a specific clinical line of research.

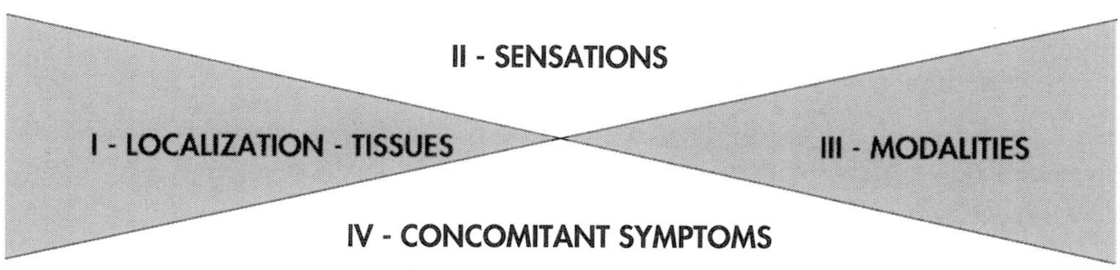

The left-hand quadrant (I) refers to the localization of the pathologic phenomena or the tissue affected.

The upper quadrant (II) corresponds to the sensations felt by the patient as a result of his illness.

The right-hand quadrant (III) is concerned with the modalities of these sensations.

The lower quadrant (IV) brings together the concomitant symptoms of the complaint in question, i.e. those which appeared at the same time as the complaint but have no obvious physiopathologic correlation.

Quadrants I and II, in fact, correspond to **conventional semiology**: they include the clinical factors which point to the nosologic diagnosis.

Quadrants III and IV correspond to **homeopathic semiology** which defines the particular reactive mode of the patient during his illness or, if one prefers, "**the clinical form peculiar to the patient**" which determines the choice of the specific homeopathic remedy or remedies.

To these four areas of research must be added, where possible, **the etiology**, i.e. the study of the immediate causes of the pathologic condition responsible for provoking the current or recent symptoms.

Let us now study each part of the clinical examination in turn.

QUADRANT I: LOCALIZATION OF THE PATHOLOGIC PHENOMENA

In modern terms we are dealing here with the **objective signs** and **pathological anatomy**. They are essential for specifying the nosologic diagnosis, but also fundamental to the homeopathic practitioner.

Indeed, we have seen to some extent from the brief study of the provings of some remedies for fever that there are pharmacodynamic substances with an affinity for certain tissues, organs, and functions, and other substances whose toxic action produces anatomic lesions; these lesions are characteristic of the substances but also similar to the pathognomonic lesions of certain complaints. This led us to emphasize the fact that the homeopathic remedy is sometimes specific, notably in acute pathology,

- to the **localization of an inflammation or lesion**,
- to the **stage in an inflammatory process or lesion**.

His knowledge of tissues, organs, and functions affected by an acute disease will immediately suggest a certain number of remedies to the homeopathic practitioner. Consequently, for example:

Ruta graveolens has an affinity for the articular ligaments: it is indicated for sprains.

Vipera has an affinity for the veins in the lower members: it is indicated for local periphlebitis.

Aesculus hippocastanum is specific to an attack of hemorrhoids, and *Hamamelis* has an affinity for the venous system.

Belladonna often corresponds to reactions of dryness in the mucous membranes, and *Apis* is specific to edematous reactions principally caused by allergies.

Gelsemium in toxic doses provokes anatomical lesions in the anterior horns of the spinal cord which are exactly identical to the pathognomonic lesions of acute anterior poliomyelitis.

Similarly, *Phosphorus*, in toxic doses, causes, amongst other things, hepatic cytolysis lesions with changes in the transaminase, GGT, and bilirubin levels in the blood which are exactly identical to the changes encountered in acute hepatitis. It is therefore the major homeopathic remedy for acute hepatitis, whatever the cause.

A doctoral thesis in pharmacy(4) has reported scientific, experimental proof of this phenomenon and clinical experiments have shown the clinical interest of this type of therapy.

It is therefore essential to stress the importance of **anatomicopathological similarity** for the homeopathic practitioner when there is any, since pathological anatomy should be considered as the objective result of the synergy of the defense mechanisms of the affected organism.

On this count, we need to understand that **faced with the evidence of anatomicopathological similarity, the functional peculiarities of the patient will be less important** and the homeopathic practitioner's task is greatly simplified when such similarity is evident.

In practice, it can be seen that knowing which tissue is affected by the disease and the possible localization of the pathologic processes may already suggest certain remedies to the practitioner. However, the extent to which these indications are to be strictly followed or not depends on whether the anatomicopathological similarity is:

- **functional and transitory** during the progression of the acute stage: *Belladonna* for dry mucous membranes, *Apis* for edematous reactions, etc.;
- **localized by affinity for a particular tissue or organ**: *Bryonia* and *Apis* have an elective action on the exudation of the serous membrane, which justifies their almost systematic prescription in cases of hydrarthrosis, pleuritis, peritoneal reaction, edematous cerebromeningeal attacks, etc.;
- or **pathognomonic of a disease and a remedy**: *Phosphorus* for acute hepatitis.

We shall see later that this hierarchy may result in adjustments in the dosage of the prescription.

Except for cases in which **the existence of anatomical similarity blurs the functional peculiarities of the patient**, the homeopathic practitioner should continue his casetaking with the study of the sensations.

(4) Bildet J., thesis, *Etudes de l'action de différentes dilutions homéopathiques de phosphore blanc sur l'hépatite toxique du rat*, Bordeaux, France, 1975.

QUADRANT II: THE SENSATIONS

This corresponds in conventional semiology to the **subjective functional and general symptoms**:

- pain,
- general sensory sensitivity,
- paresthesia,
- pruritus,
- fever,
- fatigue, etc.

The pains themselves, depending on their type, may sometimes indicate a particular remedy:

Arsenicum album for burning pains "like hot embers";

Belladonna for throbbing pains;

Bryonia for nagging pains;

Colocynthis for cramp-like, spasmodic pains which begin and end suddenly;

Arnica for contusion- or bruise-type pains.

General hypersensitivity to noise, smells, contact, light, cold, heat, etc. can also direct the practitioner to the suitable remedy.

Throughout the nineteenth century, when clinical semiology was founded essentially on subjective signs, authors described a variety of pains: piercing, prickly, biting, gnawing, shooting, boring, scraping, etc. and multiple sensations such as formication, numbness, tickling, stickiness, etc. All these descriptions are still to be found in certain handbooks of materia medica and most repertories.

In actual fact, these purely subjective, subtle nuances are too imprecise to indicate a remedy to the practitioner and the patients, moreover, are unable to describe them reliably.

These **subjective symptoms** are therefore only important if the site is clearly stated (quadrant I) and if they are supplemented by more extensive information on homeopathic semiology from quadrants III and IV.

QUADRANT III: THE MODALITIES

By definition, a modality is not a symptom but a **qualification specific to the individual person**.

It specifies a change in a symptom or in the patient viewed in his entirety; this change may be an improvement or an aggravation due to external circumstances or physiological circumstances.

A modality is always characteristic.

The following points must therefore be ascertained in the casetaking.

1. THE MODALITIES RELATED TO THE SURROUNDINGS

- **Influence of the heat and the cold**; e.g.
  - the pains associated with *Hepar sulphur, Arsenicum album,* and *Bryonia* are relieved by local heat;
  - the burning pains associated with *Apis* are relieved by cold.
- **Influence of external circumstances**; e.g.
  - *Nux vomica* and *Hepar sulphur* patients are generally sensitive to cold and their condition is aggravated by drafts;
  - *Belladonna* patients are hypersensitive to noise, light, and jolts;
  - *Arsenicum album* patients seek warmth even if they are suffering from burning pains.

2. THE MODALITIES OF RHYTHM

These are very important in the indication of a remedy, hence the importance of the timing of certain symptoms:

- a worsening between the times of one and three in the morning points to *Arsenicum album* whether for fever, pain, or the agitation of the patient;
- a worsening between two and four in the morning indicates *Kali carbonicum* (asthma);
- the aggravation of digestive symptoms between four and eight in the evening should lead the practitioner to think of *Lycopodium.*

3. THE MODALITIES OF POSITION

- Improvement when lying:
- on the stomach: *Podophyllum,*
- on the back: *Dioscorea.*
- Improvement when bent doubled: *Colocynthis, Magnesia phosphorica.*
- Aggravation from remaining upright: *Sulphur.*
- Aggravation in a kneeling position: *Sepia.*
- Improvement in a sitting position: *Gnaphalium.*
- Aggravation from a sitting position: *Ammonium muriaticum.*

4. THE MODALITIES RELATED TO PHYSIOLOGICAL ACTIONS

- Effect of rest and movement: *Bryonia, Rhus toxicodendron*, etc.
- Effect of local pressure: *Bryonia*, etc.
- Effect of elimination (diarrhea, vomiting, suppuration, etc.): *China*, etc.
- Effect of the menstrual cycle: *Actaea racemosa* patients are aggravated during menstruation, *Lachesis* patients are alleviated by menstruation, *Lac caninum* patients are aggravated during the second part of the menstrual cycle.

5. THE PSYCHIC MODALITIES

As was emphasized earlier, it would be better to call them behavioral modalities. They have less importance in acute than in chronic pathology but in some cases they may afford an important indication provided they are concomitant with the disease in question.

For example, the capricious, angry agitation of a febrile infant, calmed by nursing, indicates *Chamomilla*.

• • • • • • • • • • • • • • •

The conditions governing the appearance and disappearance of symptoms may also be sought in this quadrant: we have already studied different remedies for fevers with sudden and progressive onset; similarly, the practitioner may be guided towards particular remedies by the nature of the occurrence and cessation of different types of pain.

QUADRANT IV: THE CONCOMITANT SYMPTOMS

These are symptoms which appear **at the same time as the disease** but which have no obvious physiopathologic connection with the nosologic diagnosis.

These symptoms play a very important part in characterizing the personal reactive mode of the patient. Indeed:

- they are a measure of the **reactive unity of the organism** since they appear **simultaneously** with the pathognomonic signs of the complaint, i.e. the symptoms which are common to all the patients with the same complaint;
- they are **characteristic of the personal reactive mode** of the patient since they are particular to him and are therefore the **clinical representation of the reaction of a particular constitution**.

The **importance** of a concomitant symptom is **enhanced** if it is qualified by a modality.

The concomitant symptoms are general symptoms which may be **objective or subjective**.

OBJECTIVE GENERAL SYMPTOMS

Signs concomitant with fever, most frequently of neurovegetative origin:
- sweating;
- pallor or vasomotor flush;
- rhythm and aspect of the pulse, etc.

Characteristics of the secretions:
- fluid, thick, purulent;
- color;
- smell.

Sleep disorders.

SUBJECTIVE GENERAL SYMPTOMS

Dietary likes and dislikes:
- whether the patient feels intense thirst or not:
  for sweet or acidic drinks,
  for hot or cold drinks;
- anorexia or bulimia.

Variations in behavior:
- aggressiveness, irritability;
- anger, agitation;
- prostration;
- crying;
- seeking of consolation or not;
- sensitivity to cold, dislike of heat.

After such analytic casetaking, the harvest of symptoms it is possible to collect may appear to be enormous and confuse the neophyte. In actual fact, it should be understood that there is a **hierarchy** of the symptoms identified, i.e. some symptoms are more important than others and ***a small number of valuable symptoms*** is sufficient to determine the choice of the homeopathic remedy or remedies.

In practice, as Denis Demarque makes perfectly clear, emphasis should be placed on that which **"in each particular clinical case is the most obvious, the most intense, the best analyzed by the patient, and the most objectively perceived by the physician"**.[(5)]

(5) In the foreword to the French edition of *Manuel de Thérapeutique Homéopathique* by C. de Boeninghausen, L.H.F., 1976.

The doctor should retain:

- **from his examination**: only the objective physical or anatomical symptoms which are characteristic of the complaint to be treated:
- **from his casetaking**: only the symptoms and the modalities clearly expressed by the patient and the general behavioral changes in the patient which are concomitant with the illness.

These few, valuable signs and symptoms can then, if necessary, be related to the study of the **triggering factors** of the acute disease, i.e. the etiology.

ETIOLOGY

The etiology is based on the **study of the recent, external factors** which are at the origin of the disease and which triggered off the personal reactive symptoms of the patient under treatment.

During the provings, some substances in toxic doses are actually able to provoke in healthy people reactive syndromes which are exactly similar to pathologic reactive syndromes of clearly identified origin. These substances may then be considered as veritable "**etiologic remedies**". It must be understood however that these remedies have **no direct relation** with the cause of the disease. They are simply "homeopathic" to this triggering cause in so far as there is a reactive similarity between their proving and the patient's reactive mode.

Consequently for:

- a disease of traumatic origin, *Arnica* would systematically be considered;
- a viral infection, *Oscillococcinum*® would be considered;
- a suppurative complaint, *Hepar sulphur* and/or *Pyrogenium;*
- a case of food poisoning, *Arsenicum album, Lycopodium*, etc.;
- a chill, *Aconitum, Belladonna, Dulcamara, Rhus toxicodendron*, etc.;
- an emotional shock, *Ignatia, Gelsemium*, etc.

• • • • • • • • • • • • • • •

Let us now consider what the physician, armed with this small number of valuable symptoms, should do to determine the homeopathic remedies for an acute disease.

CHAPTER V

DETERMINATION OF THE HOMEOPATHIC REMEDY IN ACUTE DISEASES

The term "acute disease" is applied to a complaint:

- which suddenly affects a person in good health;
- which generally has a precise cause;
- which develops quite rapidly and ends either in its cure or stabilization in the medicolegal sense of the term.

Four groups of acute diseases can be distinguished:

1. **local diseases which are clearly acute and accidental**: traumatism, local infections (whitlow, furuncle, laryngitis, bronchitis, etc.), food poisoning, etc.;
2. **essential general diseases which may or may not be epidemic**: influenza, eruptive diseases, viral hepatitis, etc.;
3. **acute general functional syndromes, accidental or fortuitous**: the after-effects of fear, anger, affective or emotive shocks;
4. **acute episodes connected with a chronic complaint**, e.g. an asthma attack. These episodes are borderline cases of acute diseases, since they are in fact acute paroxysmal accidents which occur in the context of a particular chronic, pathologic constitution.

We propose to study each of these groups in turn and evaluate the relative importance for each of the information gathered during the casetaking and examination of the patient described above, i.e. the information derived from Hering's four quadrants as well as the etiology.

ACUTE OR ACCIDENTAL LOCAL COMPLAINTS

For local complaints which are clearly acute or accidental such as sprains, whitlow, tonsillitis, bronchitis, diarrhea, etc., it is sufficient to take account of the **immediate etiology** and the **pathognomonic signs** of the complaint.

From the etiologic point of view, it has been seen that there are homeopathic remedies whose reactive modes during provings correspond to pathologic reactive modes stemming from a clearly defined cause. In such situations, the prescription may be almost systematic while remaining essentially homeopathic:

Arnica has an affinity:

- for the capillaries where it can cause hemorrhagic suffusion and
- for muscular tissue in which it causes contusion-like pains; it may be indicated for practically every case of traumatism.

Similarly:
Aconitum napellus is indicated for the effects of sudden very cold spells;
Dulcamara is indicated for the effects of cold, misty humid weather;
Rhus toxicodendron, for colds caused by humidity following strenuous physical effort;
Hepar sulphur is indicated for most suppurative processes.
For acute digestive trouble:
Nux vomica is indicated after excessive drinking;
Antimonium crudum for the effects of excessive eating, accompanied by a coated tongue and frequent burping with the smell of the food eaten;
Arsenicum album is suitable for most cases of food poisoning: canned food, shellfish (alternately with *Lycopodium*), etc.

As regards the pathognomonic signs (Hering's quadrant I), we know that there are specific remedies for an **inflammatory stage or lesion stage** or for the **localization of an inflammation and lesion** because they have a toxic or pathogenetic affinity for particular organs. Consequently, for example, we find that:

Vipera is specific to superficial phlebitis;

Rana bufo is specific to lymphangitis attacks;

Aesculus hippocastanum is specific to hemorrhoid development;

Apis is specific to edematous reactions, especially those of allergic origin;

Ruta graveolens is indicated for most sprains because of its affinity for the ligaments.

If the acute local complaint is more intense, or the patient is more sensitive, it will provoke a **more intense general reaction**. The patient will show **general symptoms**, particular sensations, whose modalities will then have to be specified (Hering's quadrants II and III):

- modalities of rhythm and timing;
- modalities of improvement or aggravation due to heat or cold, movement or rest.

Included in the concomitant signs (Hering's quadrant IV) are

- the presence or absence of thirst, pain, or sweat;
- the behavioral signs (incorrectly and traditionally called "psychic signs"); they are only to be heeded if they are **clear, pronounced, and concomitant** with the acute complaint, and if they clearly convey a **change in the person's behavior**: agitation, prostration, hallucination, obvious anxiety accompanied by fear of death. However, vague anxiety, irritation, or weariness are banal symptoms which are insignificant in the determination of the homeopathic remedy or remedies.

ESSENTIAL ACUTE GENERAL DISEASES

Whether these diseases are epidemic or not (eruptive diseases, influenza, viral hepatitis, etc.), the etiology is always very precise. But apart from the case of influenza which systematically justifies the prescription of *Oscillococcinum*®, the etiology does not allow the prescription of an etiologic remedy.

On the other hand, because of the intensity of the attack, the pathognomonic signs of the disease are clear and correspond to more or less stereotyped reactive modes which indicate a limited number of remedies (Hering's quadrants II and III). For example, most children's eruptive diseases can be treated with ten or so remedies (see under the heading "Eruptive Diseases", p. 80).

In violent epidemics, e.g. influenza, most people react in the same way; in some years influenza is of the encephalitic type and almost exclusively calls for *Gelsemium* or *Bryonia;* in other years, on the contrary, arthralgic forms predominate and require *Eupatorium perfoliatum* or *Rhus toxicodendron*.

Certain viral diseases are characterized by serious anatomicopathological lesions which occasionally reach an irreversible state. **The only remedies which can check and treat these diseases are the ones which are derived from a substance whose pharmacodynamic action is capable of producing anatomical lesions similar to those of the disease**. If prescribed before the irreversible stage is reached, they will often be able to limit the development of the disease.

This is the case with *Phosphorus* in the case of acute hepatitis. In this case a high dilution is prescribed; the presence of most of the pathogenetic signs of the remedy is not necessary because the similarity of the histologic lesions is of primary importance. The similarity should be considered as the highest since it is the result of the overall synergy of the organism's defenses.

If Hahnemann never stressed this notion, it is because histology was practically unknown in his time and he only had recourse to clinical and macroscopic anatomical toxicology.

It is essential for the student to grasp the difference between a local sign of lesion (quadrant I) which corresponds to a high degree of similarity and a local sign of function (quadrant II) which corresponds to a low degree of similarity, especially if it is unqualified and not reinforced by concomitant modalities or symptoms (quadrants III and IV).

It can therefore be seen that in the essential general diseases the etiology does not normally point towards a homeopathic remedy; the anatomicopathological signs and the general signs qualified by their modalities, if they exist, will predominate.

THE GENERAL FUNCTIONAL SYNDROMES

It may seem rather excessive to associate general functional syndromes resulting from a fright, a bout of anger, an upset, or diverse affective shocks with acute diseases. Whether accidental or fortuitous, they nonetheless constitute very uncomfortable syndromes for those people who develop them and they may even be at the root of real acute, subacute, and chronic diseases when they occur in people with a susceptible sensitive constitution: functional disorders in different tracts, neuroendocrine disorders, eczema, reactive depressive syndromes, etc.

This is hardly surprising when we know that stress, because of its effect on the limbic system, is likely to have repercussions on the hypothalamus, and from there, to affect either the whole immune system or the whole endocrine system.

This underlines the prospective importance of our homeopathic action in this area, for the functional syndromes can be very quickly affected by our prescriptions. These prescriptions may be decided

- either as a result of the **etiology** of the general functional syndrome,
- or with reference to the **general symptoms** which make up the syndrome and which correspond to the totality of the **patient's behavioral changes following the initial stress** (quadrant IV).

Consequently:

Gelsemium is a remedy indicated following a fright or bad news. The patient appears obsessed, suffers from memory loss, shivers and is haggard, and looks numbed. He may also display accompanying symptoms of emotive diarrhea.

Ignatia is indicated following an upset or bad news. Susceptible patients are people who are hypersensitive in all the senses and inclined to hysteria-like displays whose modalities are often paradoxical.

Colocynthis can be useful after episodes of intense anger.

Staphysagria is also suitable after intense but suppressed anger, ill-received vexations, or negative reactions to failure.

Coffea is indicated for nervous conditions (agitation, insomnia), the effects of intense joy, or impatient expectation of a happy event. In fact, these different causes induce a state of nervous excitability in the patient comparable in appearance to the toxic manifestations of caffeine.

ACUTE EPISODES RELATED TO A CHRONIC DISEASE

Most of the time they do not warrant the name of acute diseases since these episodes are most frequently a paroxysmal manifestation observed in the context of an underlying chronic pathologic constitution. Besides, generally speaking, the remedies indicated by the immediate symptoms of the attack bring only temporary relief. In an asthma attack, for instance, the patient often reacts better to his constitutional remedy (taken in a high dilution during the acute episode) than to a remedy indicated by the symptoms of the moment; this proves that the disease is not acute.

On the practical level, it must be remembered that in these clinical cases the remedies indicated during acute attacks will often need to be supplemented, if they are to be effective, by the constitutional remedies (*Homeopathic Therapeutics: possibilities in chronic pathology*).

●●●●●●●●●●●●●●●

We have just seen that for the determination of the homeopathic remedy in acute diseases a **small number of important symptoms** is sufficient, but **their hierarchical ordering**, i.e. their relative importance, **varies according to the clinical form of the acute disorders to be treated**.

This goes to show that **it is pointless to try and draw up a systematic hierarchical ordering of symptoms**, as certain nineteenth century practitioners tried to do.

THE HOMEOPATHIC PHYSICIAN MUST APPLY A CLINICAL METHOD BUT SHOULD NOT BE THE PRISONER OF A DOCTRINE.

These symptoms should be looked for in the clinical information produced according to one or more of Hering's four quadrants and possibly in the knowledge of the etiology of the diseases.

●●●●●●●●●●●●●●●

To resume, the homeopathic remedy or remedies for an acute complaint are chosen according to:

1. **the immediate etiologic signs**, if there are any;
2. **the pathognomonic signs of the disease** (especially, therefore, the local signs), ***with priority accorded to the anatomicopathological similarity if there is any***;
3. **the general concomitant reactive symptoms** and possibly the signs of nervous behavior (incorrectly called "psychic signs"), if they are clear and occur at the same time as the complaint in question.

As for the **hierarchical ordering of the symptoms**, it **varies** according to the clinical case. It cannot be repeated enough that, **after the anatomicopathological signs**, the most important symptoms are those which are **the most intense, the most obvious, the ones that the patient expresses best, and the most objectively perceived by the practitioner**.

In homeopathy, as in medicine generally, **the clinical approach alone should predominate** and the determination of the acute homeopathic remedy or remedies should always be made **by taking account of the nosologic diagnosis**.

It is in fact fundamental to always bear in mind the **limits** as well as the **possibilities** of homeopathy. For a **homeopathic treatment to be possible and effective** in accordance with the basic definitions of the method, three conditions should always be fulfilled; these are as follows:

1. **the lesion to be treated is in fact reversible**;
2. **the patient is capable of reacting** and therefore his organism is able to support this reaction;
3. **a substance exists which is able to**:

- **provoke "similar suffering" in a healthy person** and
- **provoke a salutary reaction in the patient**.

●●●●●●●●●●●●●●●

CHAPTER VI

THIRD ORIGINAL FEATURE: THE HOMEOPATHIC REMEDY

The third original feature of homeopathic medicine is the use of the remedy in **extremely diluted doses**. This feature, which the general public often sees as the essence of homeopathy, is really only the corollary in terms of posology of the **phenomenon of similars**.

Indeed, if a patient were given too strong a material dose of medicine, this would imply adding medicinal intoxication to the clinical picture. Faced with the need to reduce the toxicity of the remedies to a minimum, Hahnemann had the idea of diminishing progressively the dosage of the substance used down to the infinitesimal dose; he noticed that the extreme dilution of the remedy combined with a series of **succussions** (shakes) after each new dilution, **not only diminished the toxic effect but increased the effectiveness of the medicine obtained**.

Infinitesimal dilution is therefore justified by the observation of clinical and experimental facts.

THE PRODUCTION PROCESS

Homeopathic preparations are obtained from products of botanical and biological origin (venom, etc.) and chemicals of mineral origin (*Cuprum* = copper) or organic origin (glands).

STRAINS

STRAINS OF BOTANICAL ORIGIN

Mother tinctures (MT) of botanical origin are obtained by macerating fresh plants or parts of plants and occasionally dried plants in alcohol. Maceration is carried out in glass or stainless steel containers and takes at least three weeks.

After macerating, the mother tinctures are decanted, filtered, stored in special conditions, and rigorously checked. The mass of mother tincture obtained in this way equals ten times the mass of raw material before processing (calculated in proportion to the mass of dried raw material).

STRAINS OF BIOLOGICAL ORIGIN

These are made from:

- whole living animals (*Apis mellifica* = whole bee, *Formica rufa* = red ant, etc.);
- from particular parts or organs of animals, secretions (*Sepia* = ink from the pouch of the cuttlefish), or venom (*Lachesis*).

STRAINS OF CHEMICAL ORIGIN

These are of mineral or organic origin; they consist of

- single or complex substances: metals, metalloids, hormones, vitamins;
- complex chemicals of natural or synthetic origin.

Nosodes are homeopathic attenuations of: pathological organs or tissues; causative agents such as bacteria, fungi, ova, parasites, virus particles, and yeast; disease products; excretions or secretions.

Isodes are homeopathic attenuations of botanical, zoological, or chemical substances, including drugs, excipients, or binders, which have been ingested or otherwise absorbed by the body and are believed to have produced a disease or disorder which interferes with homeostasis.

Allersodes are homeopathic attenuations of antigens, i.e. substances which, under suitable conditions, can induce the formation of antibodies.

Sarcodes are homeopathic attenuation of wholesome organs, tissues, or metabolic factors obtained from healthy specimens.

FROM MOTHER TINCTURE TO INFINITESIMAL DILUTION

The dilution is prepared from the mother tincture or from the chemical or biological strain.

The dilution operation is very delicate, hence the need to take as many precautions as possible:

- **The atmosphere must be as pure as possible**: the air in cities, even if only slightly polluted, contains traces of sulfur, mercury, lead, and other toxic substances (CO_2, etc.) in suspension which might react with the homeopathic dilutions to form complex chemicals far removed from the initial prescription. This is why a filtered air system which lowers the pollution level is used inside the laboratory.
- **The dilution operations** are carried out in a laminar flow enclosure which filters the air down to less than 100 particles for 30 liters of air (class 100 of American Federal Standard 209). A particle counter checks that the norm is respected.

This degree of air purity would be pointless if **the equipment and solvent were not also totally purified**:

- the solvent is 70 percent *V/V* alcohol;
- the flasks used for the dilutions are washed three times consecutively in water, then sterilized at 180° for an hour; these flasks, of an appropriate shape and quality, are emptied of the ambient air which is replaced with the pure air from the laminar flow enclosure.

Several types of dilution are used in homeopathy:

- **hahnemannian centesimal dilutions: C**; this is the most frequently used (1/100); it is prepared by mixing one part of the basic substance and 99 parts of the solvent; the mixture is vigorously shaken - "**potentized**" is the term used - in a vibratory device and this produces the first hahnemannian centesimal: 1C; 1 part of this first hahnemannian centesimal mixed with 99 parts of solvent gives the second C, and so on;
- **hahnemannian decimal dilutions: X**; this is a dilution to 1/10.

The homeopathic medicine is a substance which acts in infinitesimal doses and has to undergo a series of successive dilutions and "dynamizations" to acquire this property.

- **korsakovian dilution: K**; in 1832, Korsakov proposed a dilution technique known as "*the single bottle technique*": 5 ml of the mother tincture is placed in a bottle which is shaken vigorously and then emptied by suction. This process leaves 1% of the initial volume behind in the glass. Purified water is added to dilute the MT remaining on the sides of the bottle which is vigorously shaken **to produce the first korsakovian dilution: 1K**. By repeating the operation, the second korsakovian dilution is obtained, and so on.

Production is carried out using automatic apparatus which ensures the precision and repetition of the operation. This method requires many repeated operations to obtain high dilutions.

TRITURATION

If the strain is insoluble in water and alcohol, a trituration is prepared (e.g. *Cuprum* = copper).

1 part of basic substance is mixed with 99 parts of lactose in a mortar thus producing trituration 1C. If the operation is repeated trituration 2C is obtained, then 3C. A liquid dilution can be obtained from this trituration by dissolving part of it in 100 parts of solvent. This solution may then be used to produce new dilutions.

TRIPLE IMPREGNATION

Homeopathic remedies are most often presented in the form of large or small pellets impregnated with the homeopathic dilution.

These are little lactose crystals enveloped in saccharose and lactose. The envelope is produced in turbines specially designed to function continuously. It takes approximately two weeks to produce a small pellet and a few days longer for a large pellet.

It used to be the case that the impregnation of the pellets affected only the surface area which explains why it was not advisable to pick up the medicines with the fingers. In 1961, the process of **triple impregnation** was perfected by Jean Boiron; ***the improvement in the quality of the pellet and the triple impregnation using automatic processes made it possible to improve the homogeneity and the stability of the homeopathic medicine.***

THE FORM OF THE MEDICINES

Certain forms are specific to homeopathy:

- **large pellets** are packaged in tubes of 80 weighing 4g which are prescribed at every dilution in doses of five pellets;
- **small pellets**; a unit-dose tube of 1g contains about 200; it has to be taken all at once letting the contents dissolve under the tongue;
- **drops** come in the form of an excipient with 30 percent *V/V* alcohol. They are mostly used in low dilutions (X and MT) and taken either pure or diluted in neutral water.

All the other galenic forms are found in homeopathy: ointments, ampules, suppositories, vaginal suppositories, etc.

These medicines are:

- either **single remedies** which have only one component,
- or **complex remedies** which are mixtures of homeopathic single remedies with similar clinical indications.

PARTICULAR PRECAUTIONS TO BE TAKEN WITH HOMEOPATHIC MEDICINES

Because of their particular condition of dilution, homeopathic medicines are sensitive to certain volatile odorous substances; if the pellets are too near ether, camphor, or perfume, they may be altered; the tubes containing the pellets should not be heated; strong heat may actually modify the therapeutic action of the remedy.

It is advisable to take homeopathic medicines outside meal times: 10 minutes is ample time.

Contrary to popular belief, mint and coffee do not act as an antidote to the action of the medicines, provided they are not taken at the same time.

The taking of homeopathic medicines does not exclude association with other medicines, in particular allopathic medicines, as they do not act on the same level.

CHAPTER VII

POSOLOGY AND PRESCRIPTION FOR ACUTE DISEASES

Following these clarifications of the homeopathic remedy, the reader should always bear in mind certain characteristics specific to this remedy:

1. **there is never any chemical toxicity**, given the dilutions at which it is prescribed (starting from 4C and above);
2. **it does not act chemically**, but probably in relation to a **particular physical state**, linked to its mode of preparation and transmitted to the organism by means of a support which is the pharmaceutical form of the remedy;
3. **by itself, it has no pharmacodynamic power** (which explains the difficulty of statistical research on both the fundamental and clinical levels); **it is able to provoke a reaction in a sick organism - and no other** - because this organism is **sensitized** to its action through its particular reactive mode, which corresponds to the pharmacodynamic potential of the basic substance.

The homeopathic remedy is a

REGULATOR WHICH IS SPECIFIC TO THE AFFECTED ORGANISM

To use a didactic image which might clarify the process we could say that everything happens as if the affected organism reacted like a television set which can only receive and amplify the signals corresponding to the channel to which it is tuned, that is to say "sensitized". For example a patient whose pathologic reactive mode corresponds to the proving of *Belladonna* will only react to *Belladonna*. If he takes another remedy, it will have no therapeutic effect and his disease will follow its chosen course.

The homeopathic remedy acts through the phenomenon of ***qualitative reaction*** while the conventional remedy acts through the phenomenon of ***quantitative action***, that is, as a result of chemical action proportional to the mass prescribed. This is why the dosage in conventional medicine is defined by strict weight limits:

- below the lower limit, the remedy does not have any action or has an insufficient action;
- above the upper limit, it becomes toxic and even dangerous.

It is therefore essential, in chemotherapy, to respect scrupulously a dosage which is generally measured in milligrams of the medicinal substance per kilo of body weight or per unit of body surface area.

With the homeopathic remedy, which is a **reactive remedy that works in infinitesimal doses**, there is never any risk of chemical intoxication or overdose; therefore the **dosage** is always **independent of the weight and age of the patient**. It only works if it is administered in a dosage which is **above a certain limit that corresponds to the threshold of the patient's reactive sensitivity**.

This threshold, of course, varies from one person to another but as is the case with threshold phenomena, the reaction either does or does not take place; it is not proportional to the quantity of the prescribed support. The intensity of the reaction is only related to the reactive potential of the constitution in question.

Now, under present living conditions, chemical pollution, whether industrial, agricultural, or medical, has unquestionably led to a mithridatism of organisms and therefore to a raising of the threshold of reactivity in most people compared to what it may have been in earlier times.

Therefore, to be more sure of his effectiveness, it is important for the homeopath to prescribe enough of the "support", enough of the "pharmaceutical form". In fact, if it can be affirmed that the taking of two unit-dose tubes at the same time is no more effective than one alone, we can not be sure that the taking of a single pellet will be as clearly effective as taking five pellets at the same time.

This is why in practice homeopaths started prescribing **pellets in quantities of five at a time** when a remedy has to be taken **several times a day**, and **whole unit-dose tubes** when a remedy has only to be taken **once a day or less**.

Therefore, the first point to emphasize in the study of posology and prescription is:

In homeopathic medicine,

because of the absence of chemical toxicity in the remedies,

THE QUANTITY OF THE PHARMACEUTICAL FORM PRESCRIBED IS RELATIVELY SECONDARY.

As there is never any risk of chemical intoxication or overdosing, the only risk is not to prescribe enough of the pharmaceutical form and so not to pass the reactivity threshold of the organism to be treated.

If this notion was more widespread and better assimilated by the medical corps, it would prevent, as is seen too often:

- **homeopathic practitioners** from prescribing one or two pellets per day to their patients and so leaving them practically without treatment;
- **doctors ignorant** of homeopathic medicine sending young patients who have just swallowed a whole tube of a homeopathic remedy to the emergency department of the hospital.

But, if the quantity of the pharmaceutical form is of secondary importance, what really defines dosage in homeopathy?

DOSAGE IN HOMEOPATHY

In fact, this is a logical extension of the basic principle of homeopathy. Since the similarity defines a medicine which works in the same way as the global reactions of the sick organism, the medicine must be administered in a dose just strong enough to aid this reaction without aggravating it unpleasantly.

Therefore, ***the greater the similarity*** between the reactive mode of the patient and the proving of the remedy, ***the higher the dilution to use and vice-versa***.

The outcome is that **for each level of similarity there are corresponding levels of dilutions**. Let us take a concrete example. In the proving of *Belladonna*, there are:

- **local signs**: redness, pain, heat, dryness of the mucous membranes;
- **general signs and modalities**: fluctuant fever, profuse sweating, hyperesthesia to light, contact, jolts, etc.;
- **nervous signs**: alternative agitation and dejection, hallucinations, convulsions.

Faced with a patient whose reactive similarity compared with the proving of *Belladonna* is at the level of the **local signs**, the homeopathic similarity is slight. A **low dilution** is to be prescribed: 5C.

If the similarity is at the level of the **general symptoms** or the **modalities**, the homeopathic similarity is more pronounced. A medium dilution is to be prescribed:9C.

If the similarity extends to the level of the **general behavior**, to the level of the **nervous symptoms**, the clinical picture is much more serious and the homeopathic similarity, in relation to the proving, is much more complete. In this case, a **high dilution** is prescribed: 15 or 30C.

This can be summarized as follows: if the similarity is established:

- at the level of the **local signs**:
  ....➤ **prescribe a low dilution** (5C);
- at the level of the **general signs** and/or the **modalities**:
  ....➤ **prescribe a medium dilution** (9C);
- at the level of the **nervous symptoms** or **general behavior**:
  ....➤ **prescribe a high dilution** (15 or 30C).

If the determination of the remedy is based on pathological anatomy, the homeopathic similarity is also hierarchically structured since it corresponds to a reactive similarity, not only in its modalities but also its results. Depending on the particular case (extent, lability or stability of the lesion, nature of the tissue in question, pharmacodynamic action of the basic substance), **low, medium** or **high dilutions** are prescribed. Therefore:

In homeopathy, dosage is above all the scale of dilution.

It is this which determines the quality of the reaction: local, general, or deeply-seated.

In practice, however, there is no need or justification to use the whole, theoretically possible, range of dilutions, from the mother tincture to 30C. It is generally agreed that the higher the dilution the more comprehensive is the dilution level. It is clinically impossible to distinguish the action between 9C and 10C, between 14C and 15C, and even less so, between 27C and 30C.

For this reason, we advise you to confine your prescriptions to the dilution levels indicated earlier to facilitate the task of the pharmacist (it would be impossible for him to stock all the pharmaceutical forms at every dilution) and, consequently, avoid any delay in the supply of your patient's prescription.

But, since the homeopathic remedy is a specific stimulant of the affected organism,

Dosage is also the repeated taking of the remedies.

In an acute disease, **the action of the medicines declines in proportion to the intensity of the disease**.

The remedies are prescribed, therefore, to be taken from several times a day to several times an hour depending on the case.

In laryngitis stridulosa for example, the administration of the remedies may be justified every 5 to 10 minutes, in time with the fits of barking coughing.

For an acute febrile condition, the remedies are prescribed every hour or every two, three, or four hours, depending on the acuteness of the fever.

When **several remedies** are indicated for the same patient **they should be taken alternately** rather than together. Given what was said about dilutions, there is a risk in fact that the mixture of the dilutions of two remedies may change their particular physical state and alter their therapeutic potential. This is especially true for medium and high dilutions.

It is always the clinical condition which should guide the practitioner and in any case **the doses will be taken at longer intervals depending on the improvement in the clinical condition of the patient**.

In certain older books on homeopathy, the authors tried to give a didactic analysis of posology in stating:

- that low dilutions were reserved for acute diseases and had a short, superficial action;
- that medium dilutions were more suitable for subacute and chronic cases and ought to be only administered once or twice a day;
- that high dilutions were reserved for chronic cases and should only be prescribed very occasionally because of their deep, long-lasting action.

These distinctions are much too simplistic and arbitrary. Given our present state of knowledge, directives other than those we have indicated cannot be given without adopting a biased position for a presumed mode of action of our dilutions.

It must be understood that we can never presume with any certainty, the remedy being reactive, that we shall obtain a particular reaction since, for every patient, this reaction always depends on three factors:

- the patient,
- the disease,
- the medicine.

In some cases, a remedy which is strongly homeopathic to the reactive mode will react with a particular patient in any dilution.

In other cases, a particular patient will only be sensitive to medium dilutions or high dilutions, or a particular remedy will be more reliable used at one level of dilution than another.

Often, the remedies which provoke discharges (serous, mucous, or purulent) in their provings exhibit a different effect according to the dilution used:

- low dilutions encourage discharges;
- high dilutions slow them down or dry them up.

It can be seen therefore that it is impossible to systematize and give strict rules. Such rules, besides, would be totally unjustified practically and intellectually for they might lead one to think that, through their dereliction, the patient may be put at risk when in fact the homeopathic remedy is always **chemically non-toxic**.

It should also be known that in an acute disease, especially a febrile one, the transitory exaggeration of a few symptoms, e.g. the fever, may be observed at the beginning of the treatment. This is normal since we are acting through our prescription in the same way as the defense of the organism. This pseudo-aggravation does not last more than a few hours; it is quickly followed by a feeling of improved well-being which is of excellent prognosis.

•••••••••••••••

To summarize the question of posology for acute diseases, let us say there are three principal lines of force to respect.

1. THE HOMEOPATHIC MEDICINE

- is a **specific regulator of the organism, always chemically non-toxic**;
- it acts in relation to a **particular physical state** which is the result of its method of preparation and is best conveyed to the organism by sublingual means. It is therefore necessary to look for the pharmaceutical forms which afford the **maximum surface effect** and which can be prepared in advance and easily stored by the pharmacist to facilitate fast delivery of prescriptions;
- the **unit-dose tube of small pellets** is the preferred form. It is used for medicines which have to be taken less than once a day or once a day for a limited period;
- **large pellets** are next. They are to be used when the medicine has to be taken several times a day or once a day over long periods.

2. TWO MAJOR FUNDAMENTAL PRINCIPLES

- **The greater the similarity, the higher the dilution to be used and, conversely, the lesser the similarity, the lower the dilution.**
- **The medicine should be taken less frequently as the clinical state of the patient improves.**

3. ONLY USE PARTICULAR LEVELS OF DILUTIONS

- **5C for low dilutions;**
- **9C for medium dilutions;**
- **15 or 30C for high dilutions.**

Remember that these indications are only general directives which are not in the least absolute. Ultimately, they will remain very flexible since homeopathic medicine, chemically non-toxic, is always a function of three variables, the patient, the disease, and the remedy, and since the reactive margin of an organism is all the wider as the medicine is well chosen.

You will become progressively more familiar with all the nuances of posology, which come with practice, by studying the second part of this book in which for each clinical case we specify the dosage which has always seemed to us to be the most reliable.

PART TWO

CLINICAL APPLICATIONS

CHAPTER I

INFECTIOUS PATHOLOGY

INFLUENZA WITHOUT COMPLICATIONS AND INFLUENZAL SYNDROMES

Influenza is a contagious viral disease caused by an influenza myxovirus; there are three known types: A, B, and C and several strains. Although immunity to this virus is conferred by the secretion of antibodies against the viral surface antigen, the same person can display the symptoms of influenza several times during his life, because the virus is subject to antigenic shifts during replication and also because there is no cross immunity between different strains.

This disease occurs in epidemics; type A myxovirus have sometimes caused real pandemics, some of which are still remembered: the 1918 epidemic of Spanish influenza, the Asian influenza epidemic of 1957-1958, or Hong Kong influenza of 1968. Other viruses, myxoviruses, adenoviruses, enteroviruses of the ECHO group are responsible for very similar clinical pictures called "influenzal syndromes".

When a person is infected, the spontaneous clinical manifestation of the infectious disease has the following successive characteristics:

1. **a silent incubation period** that lasts 2 to 5 days;
2. **a sudden short febrile invasion**, with shivering, facial congestion, and/or myalgia;
3. **a fully-declared phase** lasting several days with fever and tachycardia, sweating, severe headache sometimes with photophobia, myalgia, catarrh in the ENT area, and diminished sthenia. In most cases, there are two stages in the fully-declared phase; there can be respiratory, laryngeal, digestive, pericardial, and/or neurologic complications during this phase;
4. **a defervescent phase** often with a persistent cough;
5. **a convalescent period** with asthenia of variable duration, up to several weeks long.

When homeopathic therapy is used for acute conditions, the different phases of the infectious disease are shortened, and this is even more obvious if the treatment is started early. Recovery is particularly fast when the medicines are taken at the onset of the disease. The infected person's reactions cause the infectious syndrome to disappear in a few hours. In view of the propagation of influenza as an epidemic, people who have not yet been affected should be protected and advised to take an easy-to-follow **preventive homeopathic treatment.**

The range of homeopathic medicines used varies according to when therapy is started, and in the following paragraphs the remedies are listed in relation to the stage the disease has reached when the patient is first examined.

INCUBATION PHASE

This phase is clinically silent; if there is a risk of contagion,

Oscillococcinum®

should be prescribed: one initial dose, repeated twice at six-hour intervals (three doses in all).

This medicine is prepared from an aseptic filtered autolysate obtained from the heart and liver of Muscovy duck; its high **amino acid** content is probably the reason for the potentiation of the body's defense mechanisms against infectious agents in general, and viruses in particular.

In almost all cases, therefore, the influenzal syndrome will not develop.

INVASION PHASE

This may be sudden or progressive.

A. SUDDEN INVASION PHASE

This is characterized by the development of an acute febrile syndrome, and a choice has to be made between *Aconitum* and *Belladonna*.

Aconitum napellus

Pathogenetic tests with aconite cause **shivering**, then **marked hyperthermia** of very rapid onset, with **irritability of the heart**, **red, warm, dry skin, intense thirst** (for cold water), and **sthenic agitation**. This clinical picture often occurs after a sudden chill; it tends to start during the night (around midnight or one in the morning) and the patient wakes up feeling rather anxious. A **reflex otalgia** and cough may be observed.

Prescribe in medium dilutions, 9C, as local and general symptoms coexist, in either one dose, or five pellets every half-hour or every hour until sweating occurs, which is then the indication for

Belladonna

Pathogenetic tests with belladonna cause relapsing **hyperthermia** of very rapid onset, irritability of the heart and **cephalic congestion** accompanied by throbbing pains, **red and radiant warm skin, sweating particularly of the face**. There is also **intense thirst** because of dryness of the mouth and mucous membranes (sometimes dysphagia), **photophobia** due to mydriasis, **sensorial hyperesthesia** (to noise, touch, and jolts), and agitation possibly with delirium or dejection.

In practice, the pathogenetic picture of *Belladonna* is very similar to that of *Aconitum*, the difference being essentially the presence of sweating, so *Belladonna* is indicated after *Aconitum* at the first sign of sweating.

Prescribe *Belladonna 9C* as there are both local and general symptoms, five pellets every hour approximately. Progressively increase the interval between doses as symptoms improve.

B. PROGRESSIVE INVASION PHASE

The characteristic of this phase is generally at first a feeling of faintness, with shivering, headache, myalgia, cough.

Oscillococcinum® should be prescribed, one dose as soon as possible, repeated six and twelve hours later; the first dose should be followed one hour later by *Sulphur*, one unit-dose in 15 or 30 C. If another dilution is used, **it is imperative to check that the eardrums are intact** (notably with children). *Sulphur* in low dilutions may induce the development of subjacent otitis.

The invasion phase is the last stage in which it is possible to diminish the symptoms within a few hours; we emphasize the importance of starting homeopathic treatment as soon as the first symptoms appear.

FULLY-DECLARED PHASE

The patient has not taken any homeopathic medicine during the phase of invasion and the influenzal syndrome has set in. Depending on the symptoms displayed by the patient, choose from the following medicines.

Gelsemium

This medicine is indicated for patients with an adynamic febrile syndrome, **high fever** with a progressive onset, frontal and occipital **headache**, numbness, **shivering** and even **tremor** followed by **sweating**.

This kind of febrile patient is not thirsty; he complains of fatigue and **myalgia** and his face may be crimson.

Prescribe five pellets in 9C every hour or every two hours depending on how serious the condition is. Increase the interval as symptoms improve.

Rhus toxicodendron

This remedy is indicated for patients with an adynamic febrile condition, a **high fever** with a progressive onset, accompanied by **myalgia** and **periarticular pains** with stiffening which is relieved with movement; the modality of improvement by movement is characteristic of this particular proving, and the patient has to move continually about in bed but is unable to find a comfortable position. The patient **seeks warmth**, buries himself under the blankets, sweats profusely, **shivers or coughs** as soon as he is uncovered and feels as if icy water has been poured over him.

He experiences **intense thirst** for cold water or milk. The tip of the tongue is red and there is sometimes an outbreak of **herpes around the mouth**. In this case, prescribe *Rhus toxicodendron* in 15C; in other cases, prescribe the same dosage as for *Gelsemium*.

Eupatorium perfoliatum

Remedy for an adynamic febrile syndrome with **muscular and osseous pain**, headache, and above all **ocular pain, aggravated by pressure on the eyeballs**. These symptoms are often accompanied by rhinitis and tracheobronchial cough which is worse at night when the patient is lying on his back, breathing in cold air. The patient craves cold water.

Same dosage.

∘∘∘∘∘∘∘∘∘

These three medicines have provings that often include all the symptoms of influenza; it is therefore logical and effective to prescribe them to the same patient, alternating them regularly every hour or every two hours depending on the severity of the symptoms.

However, as the influenzal syndrome progresses, different clinical pictures requiring other medicines may be observed.

Bryonia alba

This remedy is indicated for **continuous or remittent febrile conditions**, with **headache, myalgia, articular pain,** and a **dry, tracheal cough**.

All these symptoms are **aggravated by movement** and the patient has to lie still in bed, holding his chest during coughing fits. Perspiration is oily and there is **intense thirst** with a bitter taste in the mouth.

Prescribe five pellets in 9C every hour or every two hours.

Ferrum phosphoricum

This remedy is used when **the fever is not very high**. The face is alternately pale and flushed, the skin is moist.

There is a **hemorrhagic tendency** - **epistaxis** occurs - and a tendency for local congestive phenomena: **otalgia** with inflammation of the eardrums or a **tracheitis cough**.

Same dosage; no more than twice daily in the case of otalgia.

Pyrogenium

This nosode is indicated when there is a febrile syndrome and when **pulse and temperature are dissociated** (most frequently a fast pulse for a moderate fever). The patient suffers from myalgia, needs to change position with the impression that the bed is too hard. His breath is fetid and he is extremely thirsty.

Prescribe five pellets in 9C morning and evening.

Baptisia tinctoria

There is an adynamic febrile condition accompanied by **mental confusion** (or delirium) and the **digestive tract** is affected: fetid breath and diarrhea, and intense thirst. The right iliac fossa is sensitive with a rumbling caecum.

This medicine is particularly indicated when the influenzal syndrome is associated with digestive problems.

Prescribe five pellets in 9C every hour or every two hours, depending on the severity of the symptoms; administer less frequently with improvement.

∘∘∘∘∘∘∘∘∘

When the homeopathic treatment is started during the fully-declared phase, a regression of the syndrome appears after a few days and there are no complications or pronounced post-influenzal asthenia. *Oscillococcinum®* can still be prescribed but, at this stage, treatment is far less effective and reliable than during the incubation or invasion phases.

CONVALESCENT PHASE

The patient may consult for post-influenzal asthenia; he may still have a persistent cough which will not clear up. It is then possible to stimulate the patient's reactions using the following remedies.

Sulphur iodatum

This medicine seems to encourage a reaction which relieves congestion and inflammation and which corresponds to the physiopathologic needs at the **end of acute infections**, in particular **those with an affinity for the respiratory tract**.

Prescribe five pellets of *Sulphur iodatum 9C* to be taken every evening at bedtime until symptoms disappear. When the cough persists, prescribe in addition the remedies indicated for bronchitis or pneumonopathy (see corresponding chapters p. 152 and 157). In the case of isolated post-influenzal asthenia, complement with one or several of the following remedies.

China rubra

This remedy corresponds to **physical asthenia** with pallor and hypotension; this condition is found in patients who have suffered significant loss of organic fluid (sweating or diarrhea).

Prescribe in 9C, five pellets twice a day, until the symptoms disappear (this usually takes about ten days).

Kali phosphoricum

This remedy is indicated in the case of **mental asthenia** with a lack of inclination to work as the slightest intellectual effort brings about extreme fatigue. On the other hand, the patient is **hypersensitive** and easily **irritated**.

Same dosage as for *China*; if necessary, prescribe *China* and *Kali phosphoricum* alternately.

Avena sativa

In low dilutions, this medicine has an invigorating action and stimulates the appetite. In fact, its action is more related to phytotherapy than homeopathy, but it is traditionally indicated for **post-infectious asthenia with anorexia**, often associated with *Alfalfa*.

For example, before the midday and evening meals, keep in the mouth for a moment before swallowing 20 drops of the following mixture:

Avena sativa 3X
Alfalfa 3X } ana, q.s. to 30 ml

diluted in a little pure water.

Influenzinum

This nosode is obtained from the influenza virus vaccine from the Pasteur Institute; it can be used at the **end of the treatment when influenzal sequelae persist**: persistent cough, lasting anosmia, etc.

A single unit-dose in 15C is then prescribed as an etiologic remedy.

PREVENTIVE TREATMENT

With high-risk patients, the preventive homeopathic treatment of influenza has the advantage of being chemically non-toxic.

For patients with either a chronic morbid state, or with recurrent pathological manifestations, the best preventive homeopathic treatment for influenza is the same as the treatment for the chronic disease (*Homeopathic Therapeutics: possibilities in chronic pathology*), plus a weekly or fortnightly dose of *Oscillococcinum*® throughout winter.

For other patients, prescribe *Oscillococcinum*® on its own with the same frequency.

As it stimulates the body's defense mechanisms, this preventive treatment makes it possible to extend the protection against all germs responsible for infectious diseases in winter, in particular viral infections.

ERUPTIVE DISEASES IN CHILDREN

Homeopathic medicines are not specific to a nosologic diagnosis or an aggressor (bacterium, virus, allergen), as we saw in the first part of the book. They are only specific to:

- **a stage in the inflammation**,
- **an inflammatory localization in a tissue**, or
- **a reactive mode specific** to an organism, that is to say **a constitution**.

Eruptive diseases in children (measles, German measles, chickenpox, scarlet fever, fifth disease) have totally similar clinical progressions, although they are caused by different pathogenic agents:

- a period of incubation;
- a period of invasion;
- a period of eruption;
- a period of resolution with more or less severe complications.

During each of the stages, **each patient reacts according to his own constitution, as well as to the cause of the eruptive disease**. All experienced practitioners know how difficult it can be, in a nosologic diagnosis, to establish a clinical differentiation between scarlatiniform measles and scarlet fever, between light scarlet fever and discreet measles, German measles or one of the seasonal epidemic erythematous diseases which are so difficult to classify and whose etiology is uncertain.

It is therefore logical and even inevitable for the homeopathic approach to study the treatment of eruptive diseases in children in the same chapter. Indeed, the reactive modes are more or less stereotyped for each stage of the disease. They only respond to a few remedies, and it is easy for the homeopath to choose from these the remedy or remedies corresponding to the young patient to be treated.

INCUBATION PHASE

It is always more or less clinically silent and the patient is rarely examined at this stage. There is in fact nothing serious to worry the close family.

INVASION PHASE

The main characteristic is the appearance of a febrile condition which can take on two different clinical aspects:

- either **a febrile condition with a sudden onset**, as is often, but not exclusively, the case for scarlet fever;
- or **a febrile condition with a more progressive onset**, with or without an inflammation of the upper air passages.

A certain number of homeopathic remedies are homeopathic to the different febrile reactive modes.

REMEDIES FOR A FEBRILE CONDITION WITH SUDDEN ONSET

Aconitum napellus

This remedy is indicated for **sudden pronounced hyperthermia** which often begins with shivering around midnight. **The skin is red and dry, and there is no perspiration**. The pulse is tense and cannot be pressed down. The child is **agitated, anxious, and worried. He is thirsty for large quantities of cold water.**

Prescribe five pellets of *Aconitum 9C* every hour. Everything either quickly returns to normal and it was not the invasion of an eruptive disease, or else the disease continues its progression, sweating appears, and *Belladonna* is now indicated.

Belladonna

The patient is very congested, mainly in the **head which is red and covered with sweat**. He has a high, **sometimes fluctuant** fever. **The mucous membranes are dry**, especially in the throat which is red and painful; swallowing seems to be accompanied by spasms.

The child has **photophobia due to mydriasis**. He is dejected or on the contrary agitated, delirious, and even convulsive. He is **hyperesthetic** to noise, light, jolts, touch, and hypersensitive to drafts. Despite his fever, he is sensitive to cold and wants to remain in a warm bedroom with the windows and doors closed.

Depending on similarity, prescribe in 9C five pellets every two hours. In case of febrile delirium or a known convulsive tendency, use 15 or 30C.

Apis mellifica

This remedy corresponds to a sudden fever which remains constant. It may be accompanied by:

- either **a pharyngeal inflammation**, with edema of the uvula which hangs between the two pillars like a semi-transparent bell clapper, **burning, painful, and improved by cold**,
- or **a violent headache**, with a state of stupor, a congested face, and sometimes agitation of the head which the patient rolls from side to side on the pillow.

In both cases, the patient does **not feel thirsty**. The skin is dry and warm, sometimes with alternating phases of sweating.

Prescribe in 9C, five pellets every hour; in the event of neurologic phenomena, prescribe the remedy in 15C more frequently (*Apis* acts fast but its effect is only temporary). Then increase the interval depending on improvement.

REMEDIES FOR A FEBRILE CONDITION WITH INSIDIOUS ONSET

Ferrum phosphoricum

The patient appears in this case far less sthenic than in the previous cases. **The fever is not very high**, less than 39°C. The skin is moist. The child has a **red, then pale face alternately** and is prone to **local congestive** (inflammatory otitis) or **hemorrhagic phenomena** (spit striated with blood, **epistaxis**).

Prescribe in 9C, five pellets morning and evening.

Bryonia

This remedy corresponds to febrile conditions with a constant temperature and **very dry mucous membranes**, therefore an **intense thirst for large quantities of cold water**. All the patient's symptoms (headache, cough, myalgia, etc.) **are aggravated by the slightest movement**, and this requires him to keep still in his bed.

Prescribe five pellets in 9C two to four times a day.

Gelsemium

This remedy corresponds to an **adynamic febrile condition**. But in this case prostration is not due to the fact that keeping still relieves the pain, as is the case for *Bryonia*. It is the consequence of the seriousness of the disease and the deeply affected general condition of the patient. The indications for *Gelsemium* are often found in some cases of measles when "the rash does not break out properly".

The child is **adynamic and drowsy. His face is red and congested, with an impression of numbness**. He has muscular ache and feels heavy in the legs. He **sweats profusely, shivers and shakes**. In spite of the severe febrile condition, the child **is never thirsty**.

Prescribe five pellets in 9C two to four times a day.

Mercurius solubilis

The temperature is constant, with **shivering on the surface of the skin** and sweating at night which does not bring relief. It is associated with **characteristic buccopharyngeal signs**: redness of the pharynx or pultaceous coating, cervical adenopathy, **a thick yellowish tongue which retains tooth marks on the sides**, fetid breath, abundant salivation, and intense thirst.

Prescribe in 9C, two to four times a day.

Rhus toxicodendron

This remedy is indicated in the case of high, constant fever, accompanied by **pronounced shivering** as soon as the patient is uncovered, even slightly. **Agitation and prostration alternate** because muscular pain and stiffening are **relieved by movement**. The patient feels an intense thirst for cold drinks.

Same dosage.

ERUPTIVE PHASE

During the period of eruption, **the clinical aspect of the cutaneous lesion will define the homeopathic remedy**.

To facilitate the eruption, it is a good idea to prescribe systematically a single dose of *Sulphur 9C* (if the child is asthenic, a dose of *Sulphur iodatum 9C*) **after having checked that the eardrums are intact**. *Sulphur* and *Sulphur iodatum* are remedies which induce cutaneous eruptions; **never prescribe them in low dilutions** (5C), as they could then aggravate inflammatory or suppurative processes and are therefore contraindicated in the case of underlying or incubating otitis. Medium or high dilutions are used to avoid this inconvenience. Besides, these remedies have often been prescribed during the phase of invasion "to clarify the case", accelerating the outbreak of the eruption and the exact nosologic diagnosis. We will now study the principal homeopathic remedies during this phase, in relation to the nosologic diagnosis.

FOR MEASLES

At the beginning, the oculonasal catarrh requires

Euphrasia

The tears are burning, the conjunctiva is red, and the nasal discharge is not very irritant. If the modalities were reversed, *Allium cepa* would be indicated.

Prescribe in 5C, two to four times a day, depending on the severity of the symptoms.

During the eruption, depending on the appearance of the rash, prescribe

Belladonna

This remedy is indicated in case of **bright red exanthema**, with the usual general signs (fever, warm head, sweating, etc.).

Prescribe five pellets in 9C two to four times a day.

Pulsatilla

The **exanthema is rather pinkish**, and the general signs more discreet than previously, but the catarrhal symptoms of the mucous membranes are clear. **Lack of thirst** (the *Belladonna* patient may or may not be thirsty).

Prescribe in 15C (lower dilutions may induce otitic phenomena), five pellets two to four times a day. Increase the interval as symptoms improve.

FOR GERMAN MEASLES

The rash is macular, the elements are paler than in the case of measles but are sometimes grouped, giving a diffuse, scarlatiniform aspect. The disease usually corresponds to the proving of *Pulsatilla* (light red exanthema, no general signs), less often to that of *Belladonna*.

Same dosage as for measles.

FOR SCARLET FEVER AND SCARLATINIFORM ERUPTIONS

If it is not properly treated, scarlet fever may lead to severe complications (nephritis, acute rheumatic fever, etc.).

In the case of a scarlatiniform eruption, a swab of the throat must be taken. The homeopathic remedy or remedies corresponding to the symptoms will be prescribed while waiting for the results. If type A streptococci are present, antibiotic therapy will have to be started, and so the organism will have time to secrete antibodies while waiting for the results from the laboratory (the risk of recurrence is thus limited). If there are no type A streptococci, only homeopathy will be used.

The homeopathic practitioner is above all a medical practitioner; he knows how to use two therapeutic tools and he must always make his choice in his patient's best interest.

Belladonna

This remedy is indicated in most cases. Its proving includes **red, warm, painful, rough skin**, with erythema that fades with vitropression. The throat is red, and the tongue is raspberry-colored.

Prescribe five pellets in 9C every two hours.

Apis mellifica

This remedy may be indicated on its own or alternately with *Belladonna* in the case of an **edematous granular rash** with a high temperature. The patient is **not thirsty** and complains of a violent headache. All his symptoms are improved by cold.

Prescribe five pellets in 9C every two hours.

Arum triphyllum

This remedy is traditionally indicated for severe scarlet fever. The throat is very red, the tongue raspberry-colored, and the body temperature is high. The patient displays painful cervical adenopathy; he is agitated, with periods of prostration, he buries his head in the pillow and chews his dry lips, sometimes to the point of bleeding. In such cases, treatment by antibiotics is nowadays indispensable.

During desquamation, *Arsenicum album* is indicated in the case of **furfuraceous desquamation**, five pellets in 9C twice a day. If desquamation **in sheet-like scales** occurs, *Arsenicum iodatum* will be prescribed instead in the same dosage. Moreover, these remedies include a renal target in their provings, which reinforces the indication for this disease.

FOR CHICKENPOX

Unlike scarlet fever, chickenpox, in most cases, has the great advantage of having a spontaneous favorable progression. Homeopathy is then indicated unreservedly. The progression of the disease is accelerated and pruritus limited.

Rhus toxicodendron

The proving of this remedy includes cutaneous lesions which are exactly similar to those of chickenpox: **small vesicles containing a transparent, clear liquid**, surrounded by a red circle. Pruritus is improved by heat.

Prescribe in 9, or 15C, two to four times a day.

Mezereum

This remedy is indicated in the later phase, if the vesicles become infected and covered with brownish or whitish crusts; thick, yellowish pus, secreted by a small subjacent ulceration exudes from beneath the crusts.

Prescribe in 5C, two to four times a day.

Antimonium tartaricum

This remedy is indicated to remove the bluish **varioliform** scars which may persist after the disappearance of the crusts on the infected vesicles.

Prescribe in 5C, five pellets on waking and at bedtime until the patient improves.

RESOLUTION PHASE

Through the administration of these medicines, eruptive diseases in children generally last a shorter time and there are no complications. To combat postinfectious asthenia, which is anyway limited in a child treated homeopathically, the prescription of one dose of *Sulphur iodatum 9* or *15C* towards the end of the progression of the disease is sufficient.

COMPLICATIONS

Complications which the practitioner may have to deal with occur mainly with children who have not been treated initially. Conventional treatment and antibiotic therapy are then justified, but remember that homeopathy can provide fast and effective help, without harmful side effects. In severe cases, it may be associated with conventional therapy, limiting the latter in intensity or length.

Measles may lead to **otitis** or **bronchopulmonary complications** (see corresponding chapters).

Scarlet fever may lead to **nephritis** with hematuria or edema; homeopathy, associated with conventional therapy, in particular *Arnica* and *Phosphorus* for cases of nephritis with hematuria, and *Apis* for nephritis with edema, may effectively help these particularly fragile patients.

MUMPS

This viral disease follows the same clinical progression as eruptive diseases in children. The phase of cutaneous eruption is simply replaced by a phase of inflammatory fluxion of the salivary glands in general, and the parotid glands in particular.

INVASION PHASE

In theory, all the remedies already studied for this phase of the eruptive diseases will also be indicated here.

In practice, the invasion of mumps is mainly insidious and progressive, and remedies like *Ferrum phosphoricum, Bryonia, Mercurius solubilis,* even *Belladonna,* will be indicated in most cases.

FLUXION PHASE

Mercurius solubilis

This medicine corresponds in practice to almost every case of mumps, since its proving includes most of the pathognomonic signs of the complaint:

- **parotitis**;
- cervical adenopathy;
- **buccopharyngeal signs:** a flabby, enlarged, swollen tongue, covered with a saburral coating which retains marks of the teeth; saliva is thick, thready, fetid;
- general signs: fever with shivering on the surface of the skin, fetid sweating which does not bring any relief.

Prescribe five pellets in 9C three to four times a day.

RESOLUTION PHASE

Pulsatilla

This is a remedy for glandular congestion and will be systematically used as parotitis regresses. The risk of glandular complications will be limited; these include orchitis, oophoritis, and mammitis, since *Pulsatilla* is one of their principal remedies.

Prescribe in 7 or 9C, five pellets twice a day for a week, followed by one dose of *Sulphur* or *Sulphur iodatum 9* or *15C* depending on whether the patient is sthenic and dislikes heat or, on the contrary, asthenic and sensitive to cold.

COMPLICATIONS OF MUMPS

They mainly consist of:

- **glandular complaints**: orchitis, oophoritis, mammitis, pancreatitis;
- **nervous complaints**: mumps meningitis.

Pathological anatomy has shown combined lesions of intense edema and cellular degenerescence in the glandular parenchyma. As far as the nervous system is concerned, tests have mainly shown lesions related to serous meningitis.

Phosphorus

The experimental action of *Phosphorus* on the glandular parenchyma is cytolytic or degenerative, which makes it a good preventive and curative remedy for pancreatic complaints.

Given the anatomicopathological similarity, prescribe in high dilution: one dose in 15C morning and evening for eight days. Then reduce according to clinical or biological improvement.

Apis mellifica

Because of its effects during experiments on the mucous and serous membranes, this remedy has a homeopathic similarity which is both clinical and anatomicopathological in meningeal syndromes.

Prescribe in 9 or 15C, five pellets two to six times a day, depending on the severity of the symptoms.

WHOOPING COUGH

Whooping cough, an epidemic disease caused by the Bordet-Gengou bacillus, is the most serious infectious disease for infants and very young children. Homeopathic treatment is very effective; it reduces the number or the intensity of the fits of coughing and prevents complications. Vaccination does not confer absolute immunity and vaccinated children can develop atypical forms which will also respond to remedies prescribed in keeping with the phenomenon of similars.

INVASION PHASE

There is catarrh in the upper air passages which is not very characteristic: coryza, dry cough, febrile condition. The remedies which are most frequently indicated in this phase are:

Allium cepa

The child displays **coryza**, with **more or less irritant lacrimation**, but clear, abundant **nasal discharge** which **excoriates the upper lip**. Coughing is hoarse and spasmodic, with a grazing pain in the larynx. It is **aggravated** in the evening and **in a warm room**.

Prescribe five pellets in 9C every two hours.

Belladonna

The onset is more sudden in this case, with a **dry**, barking **cough**, mainly at night. **The face is red, congested, covered with sweat**, and gives off heat. The temperature is generally high, the throat is red, and the eyes are bright.

Same dosage.

Ipeca

Coughing is spasmodic and suffocating, accompanied by **nausea and glairy vomiting** which does not relieve the nausea. The face is pale, the tongue is clear or lightly coated. **Epistaxis** may occur.

Prescribe five pellets in 9C three to four times a day.

•••••••••

In the past, when there was a known epidemic, children who started to cough, but who did not go into the real characteristic fits of coughing, were given two remedies depending on the incubation phase, either to clear up the disease, or to produce the symptoms of the curative remedies of the fully-declared phase: *Carbo vegetabilis* and *Sulphur*.

Carbo vegetabilis

This remedy was indicated for children of average or mediocre general condition, who were already tired out by the incubation period; one dose in 30C, on three consecutive mornings.

Sulphur

This remedy was indicated for strong, usually fit, sthenic children; one single dose in 15C.

Nowadays, patients are generally seen during the

FULLY-DECLARED PHASE

The main sign is the presence of **characteristic fits of coughing**: a spasmodic cough accompanied by jolts with a progressively faster rhythm, which leads to redness or cyanosis of the face, then a noisy inspiration (crowing sound) with a new series of jolts. After several bouts, the coughing fit finishes with the ejection of glairy, runny, transparent expectoration.

Two remedies have a similar symptomatic picture in their proving: *Drosera* and *Coccus cacti*.

Drosera

The cough is **dry, fast, tearing, spasmodic, and barking**. It occurs in fits, as if the larynx was tickled with a feather. The inspiration is wheezing, **the face is purplish-blue** during the fits which are so close together that the patient **finds it difficult to recover his breathing**. There is sometimes epistaxis or vomiting of food, then of mucus.
Coughing produces **costal and/or abdominal pain which the patient relieves with pressure of the hands**. Aggravation in the evening, after midnight, mainly around 2 a.m.
Prescribe a single dose in 30C; there is sometimes a small recrudescence of the symptoms a few hours after taking the medicine, but then improvement follows. Do not repeat the remedy as long as there is amelioration.

Coccus cacti

Fitful coughing is accompanied by a tickling of the larynx; it reaches its peak in the morning or especially in the evening between 11 and 12 p.m.; it often ends up with **abundant, whitish, runny mucus being ejected**, or hanging from each side of the mouth. Coughing is aggravated by heat and improved in a cold bedroom or by drinking a mouthful of cold water.
Prescribe in 5 or 9C, five pellets after each fit of coughing.

Arnica

The sensation of an aching thorax, due to repeated violent fits of coughing, indicates this remedy. The child does not want to be touched; he often cries before the fit, dreading the pain it will cause.
Prescribe five pellets in 9C after each fit of coughing.

Ipeca

This remedy was studied for the phase of invasion; it can also be indicated for the fully-declared phase, with an **emetic cough occurring in fits**, nausea, and epistaxis.

RESOLUTION PHASE

Corallium rubrum

Coughing is violent, **explosive**, aggravated during the night or by breathing in cool air. It appears in isolated, sudden fits, **which the patient cannot avoid**; it is often **preceded or accompanied by suffocation**. During the fit, the patient becomes very red.

Coughing is often followed by vomiting of abundant, thick mucus, which leaves the patient exhausted.

Prescribe five pellets in 5C after each fit of coughing.

Kali bichromicum

Violent coughing is in this case followed by **expectoration of thick viscous mucus, yellow or greenish-yellow, which is difficult to expel**.

Same dosage.

Pulsatilla

Coughing is **dry at night and produces phlegm during the day**, accompanied by the ejection of thick, non-irritant, yellow mucus. It is aggravated by heat and **improved by fresh air**. It is sometimes accompanied by the loss of the senses of taste and smell.

Prescribe in 15C (because of the risk of otitis with lower dilutions), five pellets twice a day. This remedy, which is very often useful at the end of whooping cough, is often prescribed with *Sulphur iodatum* to complement it: one dose in 9 or 15C for thinner, anorexic, weaker children.

COMPLICATIONS

A well-conducted homeopathic treatment should theoretically avoid them. But they will occur in children who have not been treated, or have received insufficient treatment, in three principal clinical forms:
- bronchitis;
- convulsive tendencies;
- pertussoid tics.

1. BRONCHITIS

Bronchopulmonary complications of whooping cough are relatively frequent. They are serious because they may leave sequelae, and in particular bronchial ectasia.

The homeopathic remedies of bronchial superinfection which are most often indicated are *Ipeca* and *Pulsatilla*, which have already been mentioned, as well as *Bryonia* and *Antimonium tartaricum*.

Bryonia

Coughing is **dry, painful, aggravated or caused by the slightest movement**, and by heat. It is accompanied by retrosternal or thoracic pain, **which is relieved by compressing the thorax with the hands**.

Fever is high, the patient is dejected, with sweating which brings relief. He is **intensely thirsty and tries to remain absolutely immobile**.

Prescribe in 5 or 9C, five pellets every four to six hours. Increase interval with improvement.

Antimonium tartaricum

Breathing is dyspneic and noisy, accompanied by quivering of the nostrils. **Expectoration is difficult**, and contains thick mucus. Auscultation reveals fine or moist rale.

The tongue is coated, which is not the case for *Ipeca*.

To facilitate expectoration, prescribe five pellets in 5C every four to six hours, increasing the interval with improvement.

2. CONVULSIVE TENDENCIES

They may precede encephalitis which is dangerous because of the possible sequelae. Therefore, in whooping cough patients with a marked tendency for spasmodic reactions, homeopathic treatment is only worthwhile before the convulsions appear.

Apart from *Ipeca* which has already been mentioned, two remedies are particularly useful with these patients:

Cuprum metallicum

The child displays a **dry spasmodic cough, accompanied by suffocation** and cyanosis of the face. **Improvement by drinking a sip of cold water**.

Fits of coughing may be accompanied by various spasmodic phenomena: tics or spasmodic movements of the eyelids, tension in the forearms with **a bent thumb in a tight fist**.

Prescribe in 9C, depending on the frequency of the fits of coughing.

Mephitis putorius

Suffocating spasmodic coughing which blocks expiration.

Coughing occurs in violent fits; the face is cyanosed. **Laryngeal spasm** during coughing.

Prescribe in 5C, depending on the frequency of the fits.

3. PERTUSSOID TICS

These are spasmodic, pertussoid fits of coughing, which appear in former whooping cough patients, with even the slightest infection in the upper air passages.

They can be prevented or attenuated by systematically prescribing a dose of *Pertussinum 15* or *30C*, followed by a dose of *Drosera 30C* a few hours later, during each rhinopharyngeal episode.

This prescription can usefully be applied for the coughing fits which sometimes follow the pertussis vaccination.

ABSCESSES AND ACUTE SUPPURATIVE PROCESSES

Localized suppuration is generally preceded by an **inflammatory phase** with the characteristic tetrad: tumefaction (tumor), redness (rubor), pain (dolor), heat (calor). When homeopathic treatment is started at this stage, it may **stop the progression and avoid the suppurative stage** in many cases.

Surgical incision should be undertaken without hesitation for a collected abscess, as local and general signs often improve quickly; this incision should however not be undertaken too soon, and never before the liquefaction stage.

Homeopathic treatment, if undertaken early enough, may cause an abscess in the process of formation to resorb; at a later stage, it may hasten the progression to complete maturation and to the moment of incision. Finally, once pus has been naturally and surgically drained, homeopathic treatment enables **drying up of the discharge** and helps with cicatrization.

ONSET PHASE

Belladonna

This remedy corresponds to the group of inflammation symptoms:

- **tumefaction** with rapid onset (tumor);
- **redness** of the skin, which is bright, shiny, and tense (rubor);
- throbbing **pain** (dolor);
- intense, radiating **heat**, with a burning sensation (calor).

There is no clear modality or characteristic improvement due to heat or cold, and the patient may or may not be clearly thirsty. The only general signs, if there are any, to be taken into consideration, are general hyperesthesia of the patient, fluctuant fever accompanied by cephalic congestion and dejection, and profuse sweating which brings relief.

Prescribe *Belladonna* in *9C* for this picture, five pellets every hour or every two hours, depending on the severity of the symptoms; increase interval with improvement.

Apis mellifica

This remedy corresponds to large **inflammatory edema**, especially when the infection is located in places where the subcutaneous cellular tissue is loose (eyelids, genitalia, etc.). The skin is less red and shiny than in the previous case, and is sometimes mat. The edema is **burning, stinging, and is improved by applying something cold**.

The patient may alternately sweat and display a dry skin. He is not thirsty.

Prescribe five pellets in 9C every half-hour. Administer less frequently as the condition improves. The remedy acts fast but its effect is only temporary.

Ferrum phosphoricum

This remedy is suitable for suppuration with a **slow, insidious onset**. The skin is dark pink and sweaty.

The subject is prone to **hemorrhagic phenomena**, particularly epistaxis.

Prescribe in 9C, two or three times a day. If the inflammation is situated in the ear, do not prescribe more than once or twice a day.

Rana bufo

This is the specific remedy for traces of **localized lymphangitis**. Prescribe five pellets in 5C every four hours, and increase the interval with improvement.

FULLY-DECLARED PHASE

Two remedies can be used almost systematically, but in different ways depending on whether suppuration has collected or not: *Pyrogenium* and *Hepar sulphur*.

Pyrogenium

This nosode experimentally causes a **febrile, septic condition**, accompanied by the following signs:

- **pulse and temperature are dissociated;**
- **all secretions are extremely fetid;**
- **the patient suffers from myalgia, he is agitated**, anxious, and sometimes mentally confused.

It is obviously not necessary, nor advisable, to wait for such a severe clinical picture to prescribe the remedy, which is excellent for preventing or stopping all suppurative processes. It should therefore not be prescribed when a suppurative collection is in the process of formation, as it may delay the maturation or the drainage of pus. However, if suppuration is at the draining stage, there is no risk.

Prescribe in 9C, once or twice a day.

Hepar sulphur

Experimentally and clinically, this is the specific remedy for acute suppurative processes. In the proving of this substance, the areas infected are **hyperalgesic and hypersensitive to cold and touch**. These are not essential symptoms for the prescription of the remedy, which is indicated above all by a physiopathologic similarity rather than by the reactive modalities.

It is essential to know that the therapeutic power of this medicine varies with the dilution used:

- **high dilutions (15-30C) slow down or resorb suppuration;**
- **low dilutions (5C) encourage suppuration;**
- **medium dilutions (9C) are ambivalent** and act in one direction or the other depending on the stage of suppuration and the patient's reactive tendency.

Low dilutions should therefore be used with precaution for suppuration in enclosed areas (ear, sinus, etc.). Consequently:

1. **At the very onset of a suppurative process**, it is logical to try and stop it. *Pyrogenium 9C* and *Hepar sulphur 30C* may be prescribed, one unit-dose tube of each at two-hour intervals morning and evening, until the symptoms disappear.

2. **If pus starts forming**, medium dilutions, with their ambivalent action, may certainly be used, one dose morning and evening. They may help towards resorption or suppuration. But for suppuration at the onset (abscess, phlegmon) or for more advanced but superficial suppuration (furuncle, anthrax, sty, etc.), we prefer the technique of "scaled dosage":

- start with a unit-dose tube of *Hepar sulphur 9C;*
- twelve hours later, take a unit-dose tube of *Hepar sulphur 12C;*
- twenty-four hours later, take a unit-dose tube of *Hepar sulphur 15C;*
- twenty-four hours later, take a unit-dose tube of *Hepar sulphur 30C;*
- one or two hours before taking *Hepar sulphur,* take a unit-dose tube of *Pyrogenium 9C.*

This technique gives excellent results, but it should not be used if the abscess has already collected. In this case, it slows down maturation and may cause encystment of the abscess.

3. **If the collection is complete**, and can easily be drained, prescribe *Hepar sulphur 5C,* five pellets or one dose, morning and evening, until complete maturation and subsequent incision or spontaneous drainage.

●●●●●●●●●

Other remedies may be indicated in suppurative processes during the fully-declared phase, but less frequently than the previous ones.

Mercurius solubilis

This remedy may be indicated because of the concomitant presence of **characteristic buccopharyngeal signs**: a wide, thick tongue, with tooth marks along the sides, with a thick, yellowish coating. Salivation is profuse and nauseous; the gums are spongy.

Generally, the patient is thirsty, with shivering on the surface of the skin, and is aggravated by extreme temperatures; he sweats, particularly at night, but this sweating does not provide relief.

For this remedy also, low dilutions help suppuration and high dilutions tend to resorb.

- For a patient prone to abscesses of the tonsils, *Mercurius solubilis 15C* is prescribed in the case of acute tonsillitis to avoid a possible purulent collection. Indeed, it is sometimes better to prescribe *Mercurius corrosivus* for such a patient, as the pharmacodynamic power of this drug does not include the progression towards suppuration.
- When there is a risk of dental abscess accompanied by the above-mentioned buccopharyngeal signs, prescribe five pellets of *Pyrogenium 9C* when the patient wakes up and at 5 p.m., and five pellets of *Mercurius solubilis 9* or *15C* at 10 a.m. and at bedtime, until the abscess has resorbed or the collection is ready to be incised. In the case of an intense edematous reaction, the prescription of *Apis 9C* every two hours is an effective aid. It is better to avoid using *Mercurius solubilis* in low dilutions as it tends to aggravate suppuration.

Arsenicum album

This remedy is suitable for suppuration causing **burning pain relieved by heat**, accompanied sometimes by toxicopathic signs, intense thirst, agitation and weakness alternately.

Prescribe in 9C, two to four times a day, depending on how severe the symptoms are.

Aurum muriaticum

Aurum metallicum is a remedy which is known for its **affinity for short bones**: the maxillas, the bones of the ear.

The tests for the proving of *Aurum* conducted by Hahnemann(6) included three different strains: two gold salts (one of them at least was a chloride) and gold leaf which at the beginning of the nineteenth century, as we know, contained impurities: copper, silver, arsenic, lead, etc.

Later, homeopathic usage adopted "gold obtained by precipitating a solution of gold chloride with an excess of ferrous sulfate solution; the precipitate is washed by decantation with water with a small amount of hydrochloric acid..."(7)

Nowadays, the strain *Aurum metallicum* is prepared with a gold powder of 50 μ caliber and a degree of purity of 99.99 %.

We therefore think it is logical to prescribe *Aurum muriaticum* (brown gold chloride) rather than *Aurum metallicum* (metallic gold), which is prepared from a chemically inert substance, as is commonly known, and so has no pharmacodynamic power.

Prescribe *Aurum muriaticum* in at least 9C, once a day, for dental or auricular suppuration with good drainage, generally in association with *Pyrogenium*.

Tarentula cubensis and the nosode Anthracinum

are traditionally indicated for inflammation with a suppurative tendency, with indurated, purplish-blue, hyperalgesic integument, accompanied by severe toxicopathic signs. Nowadays, they should only be prescribed as a complement to antibiotic therapy.

Lachesis

The general and local signs are similar to the previous ones. It may help in the case of **acute pain resulting from the cessation of suppuration**, in particular in cases of otitis or sinusitis.

Prescribe five pellets of *Lachesis 9* or *15C*, every two to four hours. If the purulent discharge does not start again after twelve to twenty-four hours, surgical drainage is necessary.

AFTER DRAINAGE OF THE PURULENT COLLECTION

Prescribe *Hepar sulphur 15* or *30C* once a day, in association with *Pyrogenium 9C,* until recovery.

(6) Hahnemann C.S., Reine Arzneimittellehre, 2nd edition, 1825, volume IV ; pp. 98-134
(7) J.A. Lathoud, Etudes de matière médicale médicale homéopathique, Boiron Ed. 1991, p. 152.

CHAPTER II

GENERAL PATHOLOGY

TRAUMATISMS

Traumatism is the term used to cover the full range of local and general disorders resulting from a trauma.

Trauma is the name given to all types of wounds or lesions produced in a restricted part of the organism by a violent external shock.

The principal homeopathic therapy for traumatism is:

Arnica montana

This remedy acts:

- **on the muscles and cellular tissue**: it relieves the feelings of ache and myalgia similar to those felt after physical over-exertion or contusions;
- **on the capillaries**: it improves the extravasation of blood and the ecchymoses which appear with traumatism.

In all cases of traumatism, wherever and however it occurs, *Arnica* is the remedy which should be considered and administered first. **The more quickly it is administered, the more quickly and the better it acts**: it relieves pain and prevents the forming of hematoma or accelerates the resorption of any hematoma which have begun to form.

Prescribe five pellets in 9C every 5 to 10 minutes during the first hour, then increase the interval between doses to every hour or every two hours only, according to improvement.

But depending on the **location** and the **nature** of the traumatism, other remedies exist which can usefully complement *Arnica*.

ACCORDING TO LOCATION

FOR SPRAINS

Ruta graveolens

This remedy has an affinity for the fibrous tissues, the aponeuroses, the tendons, the ligaments, and the periosteum. It is indicated in ligament traumatism with **sensations of rupture** and of bruising which is aggravated by rest and **improved by movement**: the patient feels a need to move about and to flex the traumatized articulation.

Prescribe in 5, every hour, alternating with *Arnica 9C*.

Rhus toxicodendron

This remedy also has a pathogenetic affinity for the tendons, the aponeuroses, and the periarticular tissues. It is above all indicated for the **after-effects of sprains** in conjunction with physiotherapy; the patient then suffers from the first movements but the pain decreases as the patient persists in moving. *Ruta* is better indicated for severe stages of spraining.

Prescribe *Rhus toxicodendron 9C*, five pellets four times a day during physiotherapy.

FOR FRACTURES

Arnica 9C and *China 5C*, administered alternately, will limit hemorrhaging and assist the resorption of hematoma in the period immediately following a fracture. Two remedies will subsequently assist callus formation:

Symphytum

Very intense pain resulting from a fracture or pain in the periosteum after, or during the healing of, traumatism in the bones or in the periosteum. Touching the affected area causes aggravation.

Prescribe in low dilutions: 6X or 5C three times daily.

Calcarea phosphorica

This medicine assists the formation and calcification of callus because of its metabolic action on phosphorus and calcium.

Prescribe five pellets in 9C morning and evening.

FOR POST-TRAUMATIC HYDRARTHROSIS

Two major remedies respond to the exudation of the serous membranes.

Apis mellifica

Stinging, burning pains, **improved by cold**. No thirst.

Bryonia alba

Nagging pains, **aggravated by movement and improved by local heat**. The patient is generally intensely thirsty.

Apart from cases where the patient's reactive modes are exactly the same as during the provings described, these two remedies may be prescribed alternately despite their different local and general modalities.

Such an association is not an infringement of the phenomenon of similars. On the contrary, it is in compliance with it since the phenomenon is founded on an anatomicopathological reactive similarity.

For post-traumatic hydrarthrosis, the following may be prescribed if the patient does not display a precise clinical modality, for example:

- *Arnica 9C*, one dose on awakening and on going to bed;
- *Apis 9C* and *Bryonia 9C*, five pellets alternately every hour during the day; increase interval with improvement.

With this medicinal triad, hydrarthrosis can be observed to resorb in a few days in the same spectacular way as with anti-inflammatory drugs.

FOR THE EYES

Four remedies have particular indications for ocular traumatism.

Hamamelis

This remedy is specially indicated for ecchymoses or subconjunctival hemorrhaging, when the eyes are bloodshot and painful, with the characteristic sensation of bursting associated with this remedy.

Prescribe five pellets in 5C every two or three hours.

Ledum palustre

This is the remedy for a "black eye". Wild rosemary, in fact, causes blood suffusion at the level of the capillaries in toxic doses like *Arnica*, but the suffusion is more profuse and the blood is very dark. Improvement in fresh air.

Prescribe in 5C, every hour, alternately with *Arnica 9C*. Increase interval with improvement.

Symphytum

This is the remedy for traumatism of the eyeball caused by a blunt object, the soft areas remaining intact (from a tennis ball, fist, etc.).

Prescribe in 5C, every hour, alternately with *Arnica 9C*. Increase interval with improvement.

Ruta graveolens

This is the remedy for **ocular strain from exertion under artificial light**, with a sensation of burning which is improved by heat.

Prescribe five pellets in 5C morning and evening to prevent or cure ocular strain.

FOR THE NERVOUS TISSUE

Hypericum perforatum

This remedy is for traumatism of the nerves what *Arnica* is for traumatism of the muscles; acute, stinging, unbearable pain, **spreading along the course of the nerve** of the traumatized area. Aggravation by contact and jolts.

This remedy is effective for traumatism in areas which are rich in nervous fillets: finger tips, nails, dental pulp, etc.

Prescribe in 15 or 30C, five pellets every hour and more often if necessary.

Natrum sulphuricum

This medicine is specially indicated for the after-effects of cerebral or cerebral and medullary traumatism in general and for the after-effects of cranial traumatism in particular. Patients generally display headaches, vertigo, insomnia, memory disorders (syndrome of patients suffering from traumatism of the cranium) after an accident, whether there was a fracture of the cranium or not, and loss of consciousness or not.

According to some neurologists, these disorders are due to a hydrous dysmetabolism in the traumatized nervous tissue. This may be the reason for the therapeutic action of *Natrum sulphuricum* which appears to act on the metabolism of intercellular water.

Here is an example of a prescription for a patient with cranial traumatism: one dose of *Natrum sulphuricum 30C* on Sunday and one dose of *Arnica 30C* on Thursday; on all other days of the week, five pellets of *Hypericum 30C* on awakening and before going to bed over several months. Increase interval with improvement.

For the subjective syndrome of patients with cranial traumatism, remedies acting on the emotional sphere should also be considered: *Gelsemium, Ignatia, Argentum nitricum, Staphysagria, Kali phosphoricum*.

ACCORDING TO THE NATURE OF THE TRAUMATISM

BRUISES

For bruises, *Arnica* may be combined with *Hamamelis 5C* when the patient has a sensation of tension or of bursting, which is characteristic of this remedy.

Calendula

This plant, the garden marigold, belongs to the Compositae family; it is the traditional "homeopathic antiseptic". The mother tincture may be used for disinfecting small wounds, or it can be diluted for cleaning and dressing larger wounds. In this case, use for example a teaspoonful of *Calendula MT* for half a glass of boiled water or physiological salt solution.

Locally, this medicine has a very clear antiseptic, analgesic, and cicatrizing action. It can also be taken by mouth, in low dilutions (5C), five pellets every hour or every two hours, for irregular, slashed, and hyperalgesic wounds.

INSECT BITES AND STINGS

Two remedies may be prescribed for insect bites and stings.

Hypericum perforatum

This remedy has already been carefully studied. **Pain spreads along the path of the nerve** in the traumatized area.

Ledum palustre

This is the remedy for **stings which do not bleed** and for stings with **pain which remains local.** Improvement with fresh air.

Prescribe five pellets in 5C every hour or every two hours depending on the severity of the symptoms. For stings which may become septic, add a unit-dose tube of *Pyrogenium 9C* morning and evening for two or three days.

In addition, *Ledum palustre* used both internally and externally prevents and cures insect bites. Used internally, people usually sensitive to insect bites, or who always seem to get stung, surprisingly become less of a favorite target. Prescribe morning and evening, five pellets in 5C throughout the stay in an infested place.

Used externally, the application on a recent bite of a swab soaked in the following mixture:

Ledum palustre MT }
Calendula MT } ana, q.s. to 30 ml

is particularly calming.

WOUNDS CAUSED BY CUTTING TOOLS

Staphysagria

This remedy accelerates the cicatrization of neat cuts caused by a sharp instrument and, therefore, is used for the healing of surgical wounds.

Prescribe in 5C twice a day.

SUNSTROKE AND HEAT STROKE

These syndromes appear after long or careless exposure to bright sunlight, or after staying too long in an overheated place (car, warehouse, etc.).

They are identified by a general feeling of malaise with **headache, sluggishness, hyperthermia,** and sometimes **dehydration.** The last two signs indicate the severity of the syndrome in babies and young children; they should be corrected by appropriate methods (returning to a cooler place, rehydration, etc.).

The cutaneous symptoms may be burns or sunburns; the treatment for these is indicated further on.

Depending on the clinical picture, the homeopath may choose from the following remedies:

Aconitum napellus

This remedy is indicated for a congestive, clinical picture with warm, **dry**, **red skin**, fast pulse, and **intense thirst**. The onset is sudden and violent and the picture may be febrile or not.

The patient often shows signs of **anxiety** for which, if it is intense, *Aconitum ferox* is preferable.

Aconitum napellus is generally indicated. It suits young and/or sthenic people. Prescribe in 9 or 15C, five pellets every fifteen minutes; increase interval with improvement or change the remedy if the clinical picture changes.

Belladonna

The patient complains of **throbbing headache**. He has a **red** congested **face** which **sweats profusely**. There is more or less pronounced mydriasis. The patient feels burning and is **hyperesthetic** to light, noise, jolting. The pulse is fast.

In very severe cases, there may be **delirium with agitation**.

Prescribe in 9 or 15C according to homeopathic similarity. Traditionally, high dilutions are believed to prevent febrile convulsions in subjects prone to them, but other therapeutic measures should also be taken: ice-pack on the head, baths, etc.

Apis mellifica

This remedy is indicated for sunstroke with the following characteristics:

- **headache improved by applying pressure**,
- accompanied by **stupor and drowsiness**, although the patient cannot fall asleep because of the **restlessness of the head** on the pillow;
- copious sweating,
- **no thirst**;
- infrequent urination;
- the patient **spontaneously looks for a cooler environment**.

On the physiopathologic level, *Apis* corresponds to cases with a **cerebromeningeal edema**.

Prescribe five pellets in 15 or 30C every ten minutes, increasing the interval with improvement.

For *Apis*, as well as for *Belladonna*, the prescription may be also justified by the presence of the local cutaneous signs of these two remedies (see "Cutaneous Burns" page 204).

Gelsemium

The patient displays cerebral congestion here, accompanied by **numbness**, and sometimes **shaking, diplopia**, and an adynamic febrile condition. He has an intense, mainly posterior headache. **Lack of thirst**.

Prescribe in 15 or 30C, five pellets every fifteen minutes; increase interval with improvement.

Bryonia

This remedy is indicated when there is a congestive pressure headache, **aggravated by the slightest movement**, improved by absolute stillness or widely-applied pressure; the patient is dazed and he **wants to drink large amounts of cold water**; he displays oily-looking sweating which brings relief.

Prescribe five pellets in 9C every hour, increasing the interval with improvement.

Glonoinum

This remedy is indicated for **vasomotor disorders** with a sudden, violent onset, with the impression of **hot flushes** and paroxysmal, **throbbing headache**, with irritability of the heart and circulation.

These symptoms most often appear in subjects who cannot generally tolerate exposure to the sun, or in hypertensive people.

Their eyes are red and bloodshot. Improvement with coolness and with applying something cold.

Prescribe in 9C, five pellets every fifteen minutes; increase interval with improvement.

Melilotus

This remedy is indicated for sunstroke with a **throbbing headache** and cerebral and/or facial congestion, **improved by epistaxis**.

Same dosage as *Glonoinum*.

Veratrum viride

The clinical picture corresponds in this case to **cerebral congestion with a sudden onset**, with a **red face**, mydriasis, diplopia, intensely throbbing carotid arteries, and profuse and warm sweating. **The pulse is not very fast**. The subject remains still; he feels unwell and turns pale when he stands up.

Same dosage as before.

• • • • • • • • •

The remedies studied below are determined not only by the clinical aspect of the sunstroke, but mainly by the patients' **constitution** which predisposes them to sunstroke or to intolerance of heat.

Sulphur

This remedy is suitable for sunstroke in people who are usually **congestive, sthenic**, and optimistic, with a spasmodic hypertensive tendency. They do not like heat, look for a cool area, and have **intense cutaneous reactions** to the sun rays.

Prescribe a single dose in 15C in the case of sunstroke, associated with one of the previous remedies if it corresponds to the clinical picture.

Aurum metallicum

Traditionally, this remedy suits **plethoric patients** with cyanosed, dark-red faces, and with a tendency towards **hypertensive irritability.**

From the behavioral point of view, they are often anxious, depressive people who become violently angry. They also look for a cool environment, although they are sensitive to the cold generally speaking.

But for the reasons indicated on page 95, *Aurum muriaticum* is preferred to *Aurum metallicum*.

Same dosage and same comment as for *Sulphur*. Patients of the *Aurum* type often require *Veratrum viride*.

Lachesis

This remedy is often indicated for **women during the menopause** who especially dislike heat and direct exposure to the sun.

The headache is improved by epistaxis or when menstruation starts.

Same dosage.

Natrum carbonicum

This remedy is indicated for headache with asthenia and mental sluggishness because of the heat in **weak subjects who are easily fatigued** both intellectually and physically and who often suffer from **dyspeptic disorders** and **repeated sprains** because of the fragility of the ligaments.

Same dosage and same comment as for *Sulphur*.

•••••••••

ESSENTIAL FACIAL NEURALGIA

"Essential trigeminal neuralgia" or "tic douloureux" or "Trousseau's twitching" is a painful syndrome which is located in the sensitive area of one of the branches of the trigeminal nerve (usually upper maxillary) and characterized by one-sided fits of intense pain and lightning-sharp attacks of pain like stabbing with a knife or an electric shock. The fits are spontaneous or generally triggered by the stimulation of a specific mucocutaneous zone ("trigger zone"); the pain disappears completely between fits.

Essential trigeminal neuralgia can be observed generally between the age of 50 and 60, slightly more often in women than in men. It is different from the type of facial neuralgia which is symptomatic of an organic lesion: essentially neurinoma of the trigeminal nerve or of the auditory nerve, meningioma, and also multiple sclerosis.

Homeopathic therapy can offer noticeable relief to these patients who suffer greatly, but treatment must be started at the beginning of the complaint. The remedies must always be prescribed in high dilutions (15 or 30C) and repeated frequently: three or four times a day on average, but possibly every half-hour during painful paroxysms, increasing the interval between doses according to improvement.

Aconitum napellus

This remedy suits facial neuralgia at the onset, particularly **neuralgia triggered by cold**: the skin is dry and gives an impression of redness or heat. Very acute pains alternate with tingling or numbing sensations. The patient is agitated and anxious.

Belladonna

For sudden pain which **starts and ends abruptly**, is accompanied by a **sensation of local heat** and very often redness of the skin; it is **aggravated by cold air**, movement, and **jolting**.

Arsenicum album

The pain is a **burning pain like hot embers, relieved by locally applied heat**. It is **worse at night**, particularly between 1 a.m. and 3 a.m.

The patient is agitated and anxious; phases of nervousness alternate with periods of intense dejection and asthenia. The overall condition may be seriously affected: extreme weakness, rapid loss of weight, extreme sensitivity to cold, etc.

Magnesia phosphorica

The patient displays **very intense neuralgic pain which starts and finishes abruptly and is relieved by heat and pressure**. Traditionally, this remedy is particularly suitable for neuralgia located on the **right side**.

Colocynthis

This remedy experimentally causes the same symptoms as *Magnesia phosphorica* in a healthy person, so it has the same homeopathic indications; but its proving reveals a **predominantly left laterality**.

Kalmia latifolia

This remedy is indicated for **sudden, blinding, centrifugal, neuralgic pain** which progresses from the center to the periphery, seriously aggravated by movement.

Spigelia anthelmia

The neuralgia, **mainly on the left side**, is characterized by stinging, burning, very violent pain, aggravated by movement, jolting, touch, and damp cold. It is often accompanied by **irritability of the heart**.

Magnesia carbonica

The sudden, acute pains, like a flash, are generally more marked **on the left side, worse during the night, and aggravated by cold.**

Hypericum perforatum

This remedy is essentially indicated if the neuralgia is the **result of a traumatism**; there is a nagging pain which **follows exactly the path of the nerve**. It is aggravated by contact and jolts.

Mezereum

This medicine is suitable for facial neuralgia aggravated

- by touch,
- by movement,
- by the warmth of the bed,

but curiously alleviated by radiating heat.

Chamomilla

This remedy is particularly suitable for **subjects who are hypersensitive to pain**: these patients become very nervous, irascible, agitated, and sometimes rude when they are suffering. The pain is unbearable, aggravated at night and also by drinking too much coffee; it is accompanied by a sensation of local heat and numbness.

Nux vomica

This remedy is prescribed on the basis of general signs and concomitant signs (hypersensitivity to pain and irritability, digestive signs).

Cedron

This minor remedy, generally associated with one of the previous remedies, is indicated when the neuralgia occurs every day at the same precise hour with an almost chronometric regularity.

FACIAL PARALYSIS TRIGGERED BY COLD

Facial paralysis triggered by cold is an affliction of the motor and sensory nerves of one side of the face following exposure to a sudden fall in temperature (north wind for example) or long exposure to a draft (a long, fast journey in a car with the window open, for example).

It spontaneously evolves towards a more or less fast recovery, or towards more or less pronounced motor and/or dysesthetic sequelae. An ophthalmologist should regularly check the conjunctiva and the cornea as long as the blinking reflex of the eyelids does not function.

A rapid regression of the disorders may be observed with two homeopathic remedies which should be prescribed as soon as possible:

Aconitum napellus

Although the proving of this substance, already described many times in the course of this book, does not include neurologic lesions, clinical experiments have regularly shown good results with the use of *Aconitum napellus* for **facial paralysis with a sudden onset** accompanied by dysesthetic signs (hypoesthesia, paresthesia, etc.) **after exposure to cold**. There is no congestion, heat, anxiety, or agitation.

Prescribe one dose in 15 or 30C approximately every six hours for twenty-four hours.

Curare

Curare has a **fast, paralyzing action** which begins in the **face, with ptosis of the upper eyelids** and increased lacrimal secretion because of a deterioration of the nerve endings and an annihilation of the reflexes. Numbing and tingling sensations can also be reported.

Prescribe five pellets in 15 or 30C every two hours, increasing the interval between doses as symptoms regress.

• • • • • • • • •

If the patient is seen at a later stage, when the paralysis has been progressing for several days, the following medicines can be a useful addition to *Curare*.

Causticum

During the proving, this substance causes **local paralysis, with a progressive development**, accompanied by **cramp-like painful neuralgia, worse in dry cold** and at night around 3 or 4 a.m. Improvement in a warm, damp atmosphere.

Prescribe five pellets in 15 or 30C three or four times a day, until the disorders disappear.

Conium maculatum

The neurologic toxicity of poison hemlock associates paralytic disorders, sensory hyperesthesia (worse in the cold and at night), and somewhat slower mental activity.

This medicine is principally used with patients whose **persistent symptoms constitute a reactive depressive syndrome** accompanied by abulia and sensations of vertigo.

Same dosage as *Causticum*.

Thuja occidentalis

There are two main reasons for prescribing this remedy for facial paralysis:

- **neuralgic pain** or **residual dysesthesia** in addition to the modalities of the remedy;
- the patient displays the general reactive modalities of the sycotic type.

In the first case, the dosage is the same as that of *Causticum*; in the second case, prescribe a dose in 15 or 30C once or twice a week until the disorders disappear.

●●●●●●●●●

NERVOUS APPREHENSION
ACUTE REACTIVE EMOTIONAL DISORDERS

Emotion refers to the capacity of the human organism to react to physical stimulation, to changes in its organic or mental situation. It is expressed simultaneously in:

- the **mental sphere**, through an **affect** (grief, fear, anger, joy, for example);
- the **somatic sphere**, through **varied neurovegetative reactions** (vasomotor, endocrine, secretory, muscular, etc.).

By **nervous anticipation** we mean the particular case of an **irrational emotional reaction** which occurs in easily upset individuals **before a dreaded ordeal** (examination, show, etc.).

SEMIOLOGY

The semiology of acute emotional disorders is highly **polymorphic**. The following characteristics are generally found:
- **tachycardia**, arterial hyper- or hypotension;
- **redness or pallor** of the integument;
- **tensing**, muscular slackening, **shaking**. Tensing often affects the face, the pharynx and larynx, consequently modifying the respiratory amplitude and frequency with hyperventilation. This hyperventilation may then bring on an attack of tetany because of the induced gaseous alkalosis;
- **diarrhea**, colic spasms;
- **polyuria**.

As far as the diagnosis is concerned, the practitioner should;
- differentiate in the diagnosis from anxiety (where there is no precise triggering factor);
- try and understand the signifiance of this acute emotional discorder:
    - temporary reaction to a new situation,
    - onset of an underlying psychiatric disease: anxiety neurosis, border-line condition, psychosis, or depression.

HOMEOPATHIC TREATMENT

In the case of a real acute emotional disorder, homeopathy is a perfectly suitable therapeutic method, since there are several substances capable of experimentally causing this type of reaction in a healthy subject.

Gelsemium

The symptomatology of the *Gelsemium* type generally appears in situations of **nervous apprehension** or when confronted with **depressing emotions**.

The patient is **obsessed**, stricken by fear, **his memory lets him down** because he cannot concentrate. He feels a **generalized muscular fatigue**, sometimes accompanied by **shaking** or sensations of stiffness. He may complain of headache, migraine, **vertigo or fainting**, **diplopia**, the impression that his heart is going to stop if he does not move.

Very often, there is a **tendency towards diarrhea**. When the emotional reaction improves, **polyuria** may appear.

Prescribe a dose of *Gelsemium 30C* the evening before an examination and a dose on the morning of the examination.

Individuals who are particularly worried in advance will be given a weekly dose of *Gelsemium 30C* during the preceding month, with possibly five pellets of *Ignatia 9C* every morning if the symptomatology of *Ignatia* is partially or totally present.

In the case of an acute emotional disorder prescribe a dose of *Gelsemium 30C* as soon as possible, to be renewed when the therapeutic effect disappears.

Ignatia amara

The symptoms of *Ignatia* generally appear after grief, an unsuccessful love affair, a bereavement, a fright, a humiliation, or during nervous anticipation.

The patient displays a **polymorphic,** often contradictory, **varied symptomatology** and labile anxiety.

The following signs are found:
- **hyperesthesia** in all the senses;
- **palpitation, insomnia**;
- anorexia or nervous hunger;
- localized headache which feels like a nail in the skull;
- tendency towards **spasms**, with the sensation of **a lump in the throat** which comes from the stomach, **improved by sighing**, breathing deeply, or **yawning**;
- sensations of **colic spasms,** particularly in the right iliac fossa.

All these symptoms **improve significantly with distraction**.

If the clinical picture is mainly of spasms, prescribe *Ignatia 9C*, five pellets twice a day, increasing the interval with improvement. *Ignatia* is also indicated for **breath-holding spells** in young children and their prevention.

If the **clinical picture** is more **complete**, prescribe a dose in 15C to be renewed if the symptoms reappear.

Argentum nitricum

The symptomatology of *Argentum nitricum* generally appears in cases of **nervous apprehension**, fright, or **psychological strain**.

The **clinical expression** of the emotional reaction is mainly **digestive**, either in the form of **eructation** with pain in the epigastric fossa or in the form of **diarrhea**.

This symptomatology appears in **nervous, agitated subjects**, who want to get something over with even before it is begun: **nervous anticipation**.

During examinations, these subjects speak with volubility, with no logical order. They write too fast, crossing out words because they are afraid of not being able to express all the ideas as they come to their head. They complain of headache and **fatigue because of emotional strain**.

When confronted with a **predominance of digestive symptoms**, prescribe *Argentum* *nitricum 9C*, five pellets several times a day, increasing the interval with improvement.

If the **symptoms** are more **general**, prescribe a dose in 15 or 30C to be renewed when the symptoms reappear.

If the reactive mode is well-known and habitual, *Argentum nitricum* can be prescribed in the same way as *Gelsemium* as a preventive measure.

Ambra grisea

This remedy is indicated for particularly **hypersensitive, very shy subjects**. The emotional disorder is expressed by fatigue, shaking, spasms, hyperreflexia, nervous coughing, insomnia.

Prescribe one dose in 9 or15C depending on the greater or lesser extent of similarity, to be renewed if the symptoms reappear.

Moschus

This remedy is indicated when there is a **tendency towards fainting**, palpitations, a need to breathe in deeply, **nervous excitability** with uncontrollable, alternating fits of weeping and laughter.

It is particularly suitable for individuals (mostly women) with a tendency towards **theatrical behavior** which is very often linked with underlying sexual problems.

Prescribe a daily dose in 9, 15, or 30C. Increase interval with improvement.

Staphysagria

This remedy is indicated for individuals whose **psychosomatic pathologic condition** is directly linked with the emotional disorder, in particular **cystalgia, pruritus**.

The symptoms generally appear following **failure or humiliation**.

In their usual behavior the patients are:

- **easily outraged or upset**,
- **very touchy**, hypersensitive to any comment they think is directed against them.

Prescribe doses of *Staphysagria 9, 12, 15, and 30C*, on four successive mornings respectively, with a scaled dosage, and, depending on improvement, a dose of *Staphysagria 30C* from once a week to once a month.

•••••••••

TRAVEL SICKNESS

Travel sickness, or motion sickness, or seasickness is a clinical syndrome of **reflex neurovegetative origin**, with a labyrinthine departure point and a pneumogastric efferent tract. It corresponds in fact to an attack of vagotonia.

It affects passengers using various means of transport: cars, airplanes, ships. It is caused by the different movements of the vehicles which produce abnormal and unusual prompting of the semicircular canals (repeated angular accelerations because of changes of direction, bends, rolling movements) or an excitation of the **internal ear** (vertical linear accelerations, pitching, rolling, air pockets).

CLINICAL DESCRIPTION

Travel sickness is revealed in three types of disorders: behavioral, digestive, and sensory:

- **behavioral disorders**: progressive asthenia with drowsiness and even prostration, sensation of general malaise accompanied by pallor, coldness of the body, and cold sweats;
- **associated digestive disorders**: more or less profuse sialorrhea, nausea, then vomiting, possibly accompanied by fainting with a rapid thready pulse;
- **sensory disorders**: vertigo or a sensation of inebriation, sometimes with a lack of motor coordination. More or less intense headaches may also occur.

The disorders diminish and end when the movements caused by the means of transport stop.

They generally occur in susceptible individuals because of their personal constitution: **nervous fragility** (anxiety), **digestive fragility**.

When the patient's usual reactive mode in his motion sickness is known, the treatment should be started before his departure using the remedy which is homeopathic to the disorders, and repeated when the symptoms appear. But, as usual, the long-term cure of this sensitivity can only be obtained with the constitutional remedies which correspond to the patient's personal constitution.

HOMEOPATHIC THERAPY

The homeopathic materia medica indicates three major remedies which are often prescribed: *Cocculus indicus, Tabacum,* and *Borax,* and three other remedies which are less systematically prescribed: *Ipeca, Bryonia,* and *Petroleum.*

Cocculus indicus

The pathogenetic action depends mainly on its principal alkaloid, **picrotoxin**, a violent poison of the central nervous system, particularly of the vestibular branch of the eighth cranial nerve, and of the motor fibers of the spinal cord.

This remedy is indicated for nausea and vomiting with a **sensation of violent vertigo**. These symptoms may be associated with great weariness and a sensation of localized paralysis: the neck cannot support the head, the knees give way.

These symptoms are aggravated by certain types of visual excitation (unfolding scenery, waves), by strong odors (tobacco), and by lack of sleep. They are **relieved by heat**.

Tabacum

The clinical picture corresponds here to that of the real vagal attack so that this medicine is suitable for almost all the cases of motion sickness from the onset:

- **pallor**, then **sialorrhea**, cold sweats;
- **nausea** or vomiting;
- **palpitation** with vertigo and an impression of faintness.

There is sometimes concomitant diarrhea with a sensation of cold in the abdomen.

The patient feels worse from the slightest movement and from heat. He feels **better in cool air in the open,** or closing his eyes.

Borax

The characteristic modality of **aggravation by up and down movements and forward tipping movements** makes it an elective remedy for **sea sickness** and **air sickness** (vertical linear accelerations, air pockets).

Pallor, vertigo, and nausea aggravated by movement are also found.

These patients are often hypersensitive to sudden, high-pitched noises.

GENERAL DOSAGE

For hypersensitive subjects start the treatment a few days before the journey if possible, five pellets morning and evening in 9C. Take another five pellets an hour before the departure, and then in time with the symptoms. The prescription of one dose in 30C on the morning of departure sometimes produces good results.

• • • • • • • • • • • • • • •

The three other remedies correspond to a more limited degree of similarity:

Ipeca

This remedy is indicated in the case of **sialorrhea** with nausea and glairy, mucous, and copious vomiting which does not relieve the nausea. The tongue remains clear or lightly coated. **No thirst**.

Prescribe in 5C, depending on the frequency of the symptoms.

Bryonia

This remedy is indicated when nausea and vomiting are **aggravated by the slightest movement**.

Concomitant signs: bitter taste in the mouth and **intense thirst**.

Same dosage.

Petroleum

The indications for this remedy may very well relate to isopathy, since motion sickness is sometimes caused by the odor of the combustion of hydrocarbons. Its indication may have been stretched through routine; its action seems rather unreliable to us.

Traditionally, nausea and vertigo are **relieved by closing the eyes, eating, and by warmth**.

Aggravation from passive motion. The patient cannot tolerate traveling facing backwards.

Same dosage.

•••••••••

Given the importance of nervous hypersensitivity in highly-susceptible subjects, it seems much more important, as far as these last three remedies are concerned, to prescribe to these patients the remedy which corresponds to their **emotional hypersensitivity**, in 9, 15, or 30C, on the days preceding the dreaded trip.

Nux vomica

This remedy is suitable for authoritarian, hypersensitive (to odors, noise, cold, etc.), irascible subjects who display digestive disorders or are the type of patient who is sensitive to the remedy. They dislike not feeling responsible for the conditions of the journey. They suffer from motion sickness if they are passengers, but do not display any symptoms when they drive the car, steer the boat, or pilot the airplane themselves.

Prescribe in 9 or 15C, morning and evening, on the days preceding the trip.

Ignatia

This remedy corresponds to subjects who are hypersensitive to emotions and have a tendency towards spasms of the smooth muscles, but above all who display **paradoxical modalities**.

They dislike the smell of tobacco in other people, but not when they themselves are smoking. They feel unwell in comfortable vehicles, but very well in vehicles with intense jolts, etc.

Prescribe five pellets every morning in 9C, on the days preceding the trip.

Gelsemium

Remedy for fearful, emotive, shaking subjects, prone to nervous anticipation. They fear the trip and display **motor diarrhea** which is difficult to control at the time of departure.

Prescribe in 9 or 15C, in the evenings preceding the trip, sometimes combined with *Ignatia 9C* in the morning.

Argentum nitricum

This remedy, which we think is less reliable than *Gelsemium*, may be indicated for subjects who are also prone to nervous anticipation, who are often claustrophobic, and who also display motor diarrhea accompanied by a **lot of flatulence**.

Same dosage as *Gelsemium*.

Lycopodium

This remedy is well indicated for children who usually display cyclic vomiting. It is then a constitutional remedy; one dose in 9C on the day before the trip may be prescribed for example.

Coca

This remedy is indicated in the case of "**mountain sickness**"; its clinical signs are similar to those of motion sickness.

It corresponds to vertigo, palpitation, dyspnea, anxiety, and headache with a ringing noise in the ears.

Prescribe in 9C, two to four times a day, depending on the severity of the symptoms.

PRE AND POST-OPERATIVE CARE

Homeopathic therapy may be useful either on its own or in association with traditional therapy in situations before and after surgery. Except for exceptional operations, these situations are relatively stereotyped, and the patients' reactive modes are practically standardized. A codified treatment can therefore be indicated, since the remedies are mainly prescribed on the basis of anatomicopathological or physiopathologic data.

PRE-OPERATIVE CARE

ANXIETY BEFORE THE OPERATION

Anxiety is extremely unpleasant and uncomfortable for the patient; it can be reduced by the prescription of:

Gelsemium

Prescribe a dose in 15 or 30C a week before the operation and a dose on the day before, when the anxiety is expressed by a sensation of weariness, general numbness, **shaking**, and **diarrhea of emotional origin**. This anxiety may be accompanied by copious urination.

Ignatia

Prescribe five pellets in 9C every morning during the week preceding the operation when anxiety is expressed by **irritability** accompanied by hyperesthesia of all the senses and by **sighing** with the sensation of a **lump in the throat** and a desire to yawn.

There are also **contradictory, labile and fleeting, paradoxical disorders**, for example:

- nervous hunger which is not relieved by eating,
- nausea relieved by eating;
- **migraine** which feels like a **nail being driven in**;
- sudden, fleeting, erratic pains,
- disappearance of pains relating to the disease which requires the operation...

All these symptoms are **improved with distraction**.

If the symptoms lie between the indications of *Gelsemium* and *Ignatia*, alternate the two remedies.

VASCULAR PREPARATION

Arnica

This remedy is indicated every time there is traumatism in the muscular and cellular tissues, in particular when the capillaries are affected. It is a systematic remedy for traumatisms, since it combats the **traumatic shock** with its general action; it also limits **hemorrhaging**, speeds up resorption of ecchymoses and edema, and facilitates **cicatrization** with its specific action.

Prescribe systematically in 9C, five pellets every day during the week preceding the operation, then five pellets twice a day or more during the following week.

Phosphorus

This remedy prevents hemorrhaging and is systematically administered on the eve and on the morning of the operation, whether dental, ENT, or general surgery.

Prescribe two doses in 9C with a twenty-four hour interval between them.

RESPIRATORY PREPARATION

General anesthesia may be particularly dangerous for patients suffering from respiratory failure, specially when there is mucus in the bronchi.

Antimonium tartaricum

In its proving, this remedy has a predominant action on the respiratory mucous membranes, causing copious bronchial secretions with thick mucus which is difficult to expel.

Antimonium tartaricum is therefore the homeopathic remedy which is indicated for patients suffering from respiratory failure with noisy and **dyspneic respiration**, and **difficult** and even impossible **expectoration**. The cyanotic lips, the humid and bloodshot conjunctiva suggest an underlying chronic cor pulmonale.

Low dilutions (5C) **facilitate fluidity and elimination of the secretions**.

Medium and high dilutions (9-12-15C) **dry up the secretions**.

Dosage should therefore be adapted according to the effect to be obtained. Treatment should be started 10 or 14 days before the anesthesia, and continued for a long while afterwards.

Prescribe five pellets in 5C in the morning and evening before the operation, then five pellets four to six times a day after the operation with a dilution that is adapted to the clinical symptoms. As necessary, associate the traditional therapeutic tools: sloping cure, breathing exercises, aerosols, etc.

POST-OPERATIVE CARE

QUALITY OF THE CICATRIZATION

This is ensured by *Arnica* for the reasons already mentioned, and also by:

Staphysagria

This remedy accelerates the cicatrization of wounds caused by cutting tools; this obviously corresponds to the surgical situation.

Prescribe five pellets in 5C twice a day, for about two weeks.

If the patient tends to produce **keloid scars**, the following remedies are prescribed:

Graphites

Prescribe five pellets in 9C, morning and evening for a month or two. This remedy is complemented by:

Thuja

a weekly dose for the same length of time. *Thuja*, which is studied in the volume on chronic diseases, is one of the major remedies for constitutions which tend to develop constructive lesions on the skin.

POST-OPERATIVE ASTHENIA

A certain number of patients feel tired in the period following surgery because of significant loss of liquid or of anemia. This is the indication for:

China

This remedy has already been described; it corresponds in this case to patients who are always pale, weak, anemic, with hypotension, buzzing in the ears, and blurred vision.

Prescribe five pellets in 9C twice a day, complemented frequently by:

Ferrum metallicum

This remedy is indicated when iron deficiency causes **vertigo**, especially when standing up from a lying-down position. Prescribe in 5C, five pellets twice a day.

If the sideropenia is very marked, iron must obviously be provided in material doses.

Other patients display a state of anemia which really fits a picture of **reactive depression**, with accompanying insomnia, anorexia, and anxiety.

Here again, *Ignatia* and *Gelsemium* are useful because of their action on the emotional sphere, as well as

Kali phosphoricum

This remedy is indicated when there is:
- **asthenia** with **memory failure, sadness, irritability**, emotionalism, and headaches with intellectual exertion;
- **insomnia** with night fears;
- **vertigo** and dizzy spells.

These symptoms are improved by moderate movement or a slow walk, by company, or by eating.

Prescribe five pellets in 9 or 15C, morning and evening. Increase interval with improvement.

CHAPTER III

EAR, NOSE, AND THROAT RESPIRATORY TRACT

ACUTE CORYZA

A**cute coryza** is an **inflammatory rhinitis** of infectious origin, generally viral, accompanied by different types of rhinorrhea during its development. Some forms of coryza are accompanied by a febrile reaction. The spontaneous development of the complaint usually leads to recovery in one or two weeks.

It is necessary to distinguish acute coryza from spasmodic coryza which is only the acute manifestation of a chronic disease *(Homeopathic therapeutics: Possibilities in chronic pathology)*.

As in any infectious disease, we can observe a period of silent incubation after contagion, an onset phase, a fully-declared phase, and a resolution phase. The medication is different depending on the stage at which treatment begins.

INCUBATION PHASE

Although incubation is silent, taking homeopathic treatment immediately contagion is suspected (contact with an infected person, chill, etc.) often leads to the symptoms not appearing at all.

For its effectiveness against viral complaints, prescribe a unit-dose tube of *Oscillococcinum*® which should be taken as soon as there is a risk of coryza and repeat this dose twice at six-hour intervals.

PHASE OF INVASION

The phase of invasion is characterized by:

- either a **congestive phenomenon** in the nasal mucous membrane resulting in **sneezing** and a **sensation of obstruction in the nose**,
- or an **acute febrile syndrome** in addition to the local symptoms.

The phase of invasion may be of variable duration, but is often short; it precedes the fully-declared phase signaled by the presence of **rhinorrhea**.

NON-FEBRILE INVASION

Nux vomica

This remedy is used when the first symptoms of coryza consist of **sneezing bouts** accompanied by an initial sensation of a **dry nose** and **general chill** and the **impression of not being able to warm up**, even with lots of clothing or blankets.

Prescribe in 9C, since there is a mixture of local and general symptoms, in frequently repeated doses of five pellets (30 to 60 minutes between each dose).

Sticta pulmonaria

This remedy is used for a case of dry coryza where there is **pain at the bridge of the nose** which seems blocked and squeezed as if the patient was wearing a pince-nez. Try as he might, the patient cannot clear his nose; he may feel pain at the front of his head and display a dry cough.

Prescribe frequently repeated doses in 5C. The indication of this remedy ceases when the nose begins to run.

FEBRILE INVASION

We find the same homeopathic medicines as for patients displaying an acute febrile syndrome of sudden onset accompanied by dry mucous membranes.

Aconitum napellus

After shivering, the patient presents hyperthermia of very rapid onset with **irritability of the heart, a red, warm, dry skin, intense thirst** (for cold water) and **sthenic agitation** as well as a sensation of **dryness in the nasal mucous membrane** and **sneezing**.

This picture is seen in most cases following a sudden chill; otalgia is reported. The fever promptly appears about midnight or 1 a.m.

Prescribe in 9C, in doses of five pellets every half-hour until sweating occurs, at which point the indication of this medicine is replaced by that of

Belladonna

This remedy is prescribed if **dryness of the oral and nasal mucous membranes** is observed as well as an acute febrile syndrome of rapid onset with **irritability of the heart**, **cephalic congestion** accompanied by throbbing pains, a **red and radiantly warm skin that is sweaty, especially on the face**. The dryness of the mucous membranes results in **intense thirst**.

Prescribe in 9C, in doses of five pellets every hour and increase the interval between doses as the symptoms decrease in intensity.

FULLY-DECLARED PHASE

During the fully-declared phase, the homeopathic medicines are determined according to the **quality of the rhinorrhea** and the surrounding local symptoms. A chronological sequence to the discharges is very often observed: after a watery discharge, the rhinorrhea develops spontaneously into a mucous discharge and then into a mucopurulent discharge.

WATERY RHINORRHEA

Allium cepa

The first symptoms are a **prickling in the eyes** which quickly water and sneezing bouts followed by **profuse, burning watery rhinorrhea** which eventually excoriates the nostril orifices and upper lip due to the patient frequently wiping his nose. The rhinorrhea is **aggravated by heat**.

Arsenicum album

This medicine is indicated in the case of **watery rhinorrhea which is scant but very hot** and caustic on the upper lip when the person has been exposed for some time to **very sharp cold** (e.g. the north wind in winter); the symptoms **decrease when the patient warms up**.

Kali iodatum

The coryza is **watery, profuse, and irritant**; the nose is swollen and red; the eyes are watery, burning, and swollen. The symptoms are **aggravated in the cold air**. A pain in the **frontal sinuses** and a **constricted sensation at the bridge of the nose** will gradually appear.

MUCOUS RHINORRHEA

Kali sulphuricum

The secretions are **glairy, runny, profuse, and only slightly irritant**; the mucus is clear, and occasionally has a dark yellow or greenish-yellow hue. The nasal obstruction is **aggravated by heat** and improved in the fresh air. **Anosmia** and ageusia are frequently reported. Bronchial mucous rale becomes gradually more frequent; the quantity of this mucus provokes a reflex **catarrh cough** which makes the eyes shine, but expectoration is difficult and the patient tends to swallow his sputum.

Kali muriaticum

The secretions are **glairy, thick, not very profuse, and only slightly irritant**. Crusts begin to appear in the nostrils. There is pronounced **anosmia**; there is a **catarrhal cough** and **catarrh in the eustachian tube** which causes **hypoacusis** and clicking noises perceived by the patient. These symptoms are aggravated by damp, cold conditions.

Dulcamara

This medicine is indicated for catarrh in the ENT region with the sensation of a **blocked nose** and possibly a cough and hoarseness. Although this is especially a remedy for chronic diseases, the prescription of this substance is not out of place in this chapter if the etiology includes the notions of **cold and humidity** (coryza brought on by getting soaked in rainy or foggy weather).

MUCOPURULENT RHINORRHEA

Kali bichromicum

This medicine is indicated when the coryza begins with congested nostrils with a sensation of dryness and **blocked nose,** and also with the sensation of **pressure** being exerted at the bridge of the nose.

Initially fluid and profuse, the discharge quickly becomes **greenish-yellow, runny, viscous, and**

sticky. When he blows his nose the patient expels **hard, elastic, sticky lumps** which leave the nasal mucous membrane burning and raw. Staying warm brings improvement.

Mercurius solubilis

The discharge is **clearly purulent, greenish, and profuse, and excoriates** the nostril orifices; the mucous membrane is inflamed and swollen. Also observed are an increase in the sialorrhea, a tongue which retains marks of the teeth, fetid breath and profuse, burning lacrimation. The skin is moist from sweat; the patient shivers at the surface of the skin, sweats at night, and feels worse in the heat.

Hydrastis canadensis

The secretions are **thick, yellowish, very viscous and very sticky**, hardening around the nostril orifices while there is a **slow discharge in the cavum.** The patient has a sensation of nasal obstruction if he is in a warm bedroom.

•••••••••

At the mucopurulent rhinitis stage, it is very useful to complement the symptomatic homeopathic treatment with a medicine which helps the organism's defenses fight against fever and infection.

Ferrum phosphoricum

For a **slight fever** of about 38 - 38°5 accompanied by:

- nasal secretions streaked with blood,
- or a dry cough with tickling in the larynx and trachea,
- or otalgia with a pink eardrum (sometimes with redness of the pinna and the cheek on the affected side),

prescribe a daily dose of *Ferrum phosphoricum 9C* for between two to four days.

Pyrogenium

This medicine may be systematically prescribed for any localized inflammatory phenomena which tend towards suppuration and improve with the local application of heat, especially if they are accompanied by a febrile reaction.

Prescribe five pellets per day or a unit-dose tube daily of *Pyrogenium 9C* in addition to the symptomatic remedies until the symptoms clear up.

Hepar sulphur

The high dilutions of this medicine check suppurative phenomena; *Hepar sulphur* is prescribed at 15 or 30C, five pellets or a unit-dose tube per day until the superinfection clears up.

DOSAGE IN THE FULLY-DECLARED PHASE

If the normal rules of posology require the use of low dilutions when the prescription is based on local symptoms only, the **drying up of pathologic secretions** represents an exception to the rule: since low dilutions encourage secretions, it is wise not to use the remedies in question **at a dilution lower than 9C**.

These medicines can then be prescribed in doses of five pellets at approximately every two hours, increasing the interval between doses progressively as the symptoms fade. It is also important to know when to change the remedy as the quality of the discharge changes (e.g. when the mucous rhinorrhea changes into a mucopurulent rhinorrhea).

RESOLUTION PHASE

Without treatment acute coryza often tends to last for one or two weeks, during which time profuse, practically transparent rhinorrhea persists, sometimes watery and sometimes glairy, accompanied by occasional coughing. In this case the following may be indicated:

Nux vomica

This remedy is above all indicated if there are **bouts of sneezing**, especially in the **morning on awakening**. It should be prescribed in 9C, three to four times a day. The resolution phase is thus foreshortened.

Sulphur iodatum

This remedy appears to encourage a decongestant and anti-inflammatory reaction which corresponds to the physiopathologic needs encountered towards the **end of acute infections affecting the respiratory tract**.

Prescribe five pellets in 9C to be taken over a few days or else a single dose.

Pulsatilla

This medicine is normally prescribed at this stage but we only use it for this indication in high dilutions (15 or 30C) once a day for a few days only.

Lower dilutions in fact have been rejected because of the frequent phenomena of reactivating purulent otitis when the inflammation of the ENT region seems to have cleared up.

ACUTE AND SUBACUTE SINUSITIS

Acute sinusitis is an inflammation of the sinuses of the face, possibly affecting the periosteum, and accompanied soon after by **suppuration**. It is mostly observed during the progression of non-treated acute coryza of which it is a painful complication.

SYMPTOMATIC MEDICINES

BEFORE THE SUPPURATIVE PHASE

As soon as the first symptoms of acute coryza appear, the patient complains of pains at the bridge of the nose and in the frontal sinuses. The prescription of medicines which are homeopathic to the early symptoms prevents the progression towards the suppurative process.

Sticta pulmonaria

This remedy is prescribed for a **dry coryza** when the patient tries in vain to blow his nose; he presents a **pain at the bridge of the nose**, as if it was being squeezed by a pince-nez. This pain may spread to the frontal area.

Prescribe in 5C in frequently repeated doses. The indication of the remedy ceases when a discharge begins.

Kali iodatum

The symptoms begin with **watery coryza** with a profuse, **irritant** discharge. The nose becomes swollen and red, the eyes **watery, burning, and bloated**. A **pain in the frontal sinuses** and a sensation of **constriction at the bridge of the nose** appear progressively. The symptoms are aggravated in the fresh air.

Prescribe five pellets in at least 9C every hour (see "Acute Coryza", p. 122, dosage in the fully-declared phase); steadily increase the interval between doses as the symptoms diminish.

THE SUPPURATIVE PHASE

The choice of homeopathic remedy is based on the type of the discharge and its modalities.

Kali bichromicum

This medicine is indicated when the sinusitis is preceded by a coryza whose characteristics are congestion of the nostrils with a sensation of dryness, **obstruction**, and **pressure at the bridge of the nose**. These sensations persist for some time.

There is also **rhinorrhea which is mucopurulent, greenish-yellow, runny, viscous and sticky**, and often **streaked with blood**. When he blows his nose, the patient expels hard, sticky, elastic lumps leaving the nasal mucous membrane exposed and burning.

Keeping warm brings improvement in the patient's condition.

Hydrastis canadensis

The secretions are **thick, yellowish**, very **viscous** and **sticky** and harden around the nostril orifices while there is a slow discharge in the cavum. The patient has the sensation of **nasal obstruction** in a warm bedroom.

Cinnabaris

This remedy corresponds to **posterior rhinorrhea** with thready mucus which is difficult to shift. The patient feels **pains** along the **top of his nose** as if he was wearing heavy glasses. The pain may be intense, **periorbital,** and seems to shoot violently from the lacrimal duct to the temple with a **scarlet redness of the eye**.

Cinnabaris may also be indicated for ethmoid or sphenoid sinusitis.

Mercurius solubilis

The rhinorrhea is clearly **purulent, greenish, profuse and excoriates** the nostril orifices; the nasal mucous membrane is very inflamed, swollen, and painful.

Also observed are an increase in the sialorrhea, the tongue which retains marks of the teeth, and fetid breath. Profuse, burning lacrimation may also be associated with these symptoms.

The skin is moist; the patient shivers at the surface of the skin, sweats at night, and feels worse in the heat.

Mezereum

This remedy is used in the case of **burning pains in the bones of the nose and face**, or in the case of **mucopurulent rhinorrhea streaked with blood**.

The symptoms are aggravated at night, by cold, and by pressure on the painful areas. *Mezereum* and *Kali bichromicum* complement each other well.

Lachesis mutus

The prescription of this venom applies to the presence of an inflammation when the modality of **aggravation** of the symptoms is the **absence or cessation of discharge**, or when the modality is inverse: **improvement with the appearance or reappearance of the discharge**.

The characteristic left lateral dominance of the remedy is not a factor in the determination of the medicine.

Prescribe *Lachesis 9* or *15C* in doses of five pellets every two to four hours. In the case of intense pain due to cessation of the purulent rhinorrhea, the reappearance of the discharge with the administration of *Lachesis mutus* should be fast, in twelve to twenty-four hours at the most; otherwise, the patient should be referred to an ENT specialist for an operation.

SUPPURATION REMEDIES

To stop the suppurative process, the following should also be prescribed:

Pyrogenium

This medicine may be **systematically** prescribed for any localized inflammatory phenomenon accompanied by a suppurative phase and improved by the local application of heat, especially if there is also a febrile reaction.

Prescribe a daily unit-dose tube in 9C in addition to the symptomatic homeopathic medicines until the symptoms clear up.

Hepar sulphur

This medicine complements *Pyrogenium* for acute suppurative processes (see the chapter entitled "Abscesses and Acute Suppurative Processes", p 93). Low dilutions which encourage suppuration should be avoided.

The prescription of four doses "in a scale" provides a maximum of safety and results: it involves prescribing a daily dose of *Hepar sulphur* in increasing dilutions over four consecutive days: 9C the first day, 12C the second day, 15C the third day, and 30C the fourth day, with each dose preceded two hours before by a dose of *Pyrogenium* 9C.

PRESCRIPTION TECHNIQUE DURING THE SUPPURATION PHASE

Acute sinusitis is special in that it presents at some point in its progression a suppurative phase which develops in a practically enclosed cavity, which may become completely closed up if the inflammation reduces the communication lumina to the point of blocking them. The method of prescription differs according to whether the purulent secretions are profuse or scanty, or whether they have ceased altogether.

Although the normal rules of posology require the use of low dilutions when the prescription is based on local symptoms, it should be remembered that when a reaction is provoked on an organ, **low dilutions** incur an **increase in secretion** while **high dilutions** incur a **decrease**.

ACUTE SINUSITIS WITH PROFUSE SECRETION

Prescribe doses of five pellets repeated every hour, with the recommendation that the interval between doses is increased as symptoms decrease.

Do not prescribe a symptomatic medicine lower than 9C.

SUBACUTE SINUSITIS WITH SCANTY SECRETION

Doses are taken less frequently; five pellets one to three times a day until the symptoms clear up.

In cases in which the mucopurulent secretion can be effortlessly discharged from the sinuses, but in which the procedure tends to falter or not to happen smoothly, it is often advantageous to **reactivate the secretion process temporarily** with **low dilutions**.

ACUTE SINUSITIS WITH CESSATION OF THE DISCHARGE

This is the case in which *Lachesis mutus* should be used in repeated doses of five pellets. The secretions should also dry up with the prescription of symptomatic medicines in at least 9C.

EXAMPLES OF PRESCRIPTIONS

FIRST EXAMPLE

Take the case of a patient with acute frontal sinusitis accompanied by a profuse, purulent discharge and periorbital pains.

Prescription

1. For four consecutive mornings, take a unit-dose tube on awakening of
   Pyrogenium 9C (4 doses)

followed two hours later by a dose of
Hepar sulphur 9C on the first day,
Hepar sulphur 12C on the second day,
Hepar sulphur 15C on the third day,
Hepar sulphur 30C on the fourth day.

2. During the day take alternate doses approximately every hour of five pellets of
   Kali bichromicum 9C (2 multi-dose tubes)

and five pellets of
Cinnabaris 9C (2 multi-dose tubes).

Increase the interval between doses as the intensity of the symptoms decreases.

SECOND EXAMPLE

Let us suppose the patient presents a painful, persistent, maxillary sinusitis opaque to X-rays.

Prescription

1. Take for one week:

- on awakening and going to bed, five pellets of
  Kali bichromicum 5C (1 multi-dose tube);
- at noon and in the evening before meals, twenty drops of
  Hydrastis 6X (1 bottle of 30 ml),

diluted in a little pure water.

2. And for the following two weeks:

- each morning on awakening five pellets of
  Pyrogenium 9C (1 multi-dose tube);
- before the midday and evening meals, five pellets of
  Kali bichromicum 9C (2 multi-dose tubes);
- at bedtime, a unit-dose tube of
  Hepar sulphur 9C on the first evening,
  Hepar sulphur 12C on the second evening,
  Hepar sulphur 15C on the third evening,
  Hepar sulphur 30C on the fourth evening,

and on the following evenings, five pellets of
Mezereum 9C (1 multi-dose tube).

ACUTE OTITIS

The term "acute otitis" is given to a process of inflammation and/or infection

- affecting the outer and/or middle ear,
- which is triggered by a microbial agent which most often enters via the nasopharynx,
- which is capable of either progressing independently, or complicating an acute rhinopharyngeal complaint or a general infectious disease, or of instigating an infectious syndrome.

Three types of acute otitis corresponding to three degrees of progression can be distinguished:

1. **congestive otitis** in which the **inflammatory aspect** is dominant;
2. **serous otitis** governed by mechanical disorders due to the presence of **tubal catarrh in the eustachian tube**;
3. **suppurative otitis** which necessitates the removal of the **purulent collection**.

1. CONGESTIVE OTITIS

Congestive otitis is recognized by the sudden appearance of a very intense localized **pain** (manifested in infants and young children by tears and/or rubbing of the ears). The otoscopy reveals a **shining, pink eardrum** with **hypervascular** vessels of the external acoustic meatus and the upper part of the eardrum.

This congestive otitis is:

- either an isolated symptom or the initial symptom of an infectious disease,
- or a complication of febrile rhinopharyngitis or adenoiditis which is just beginning.

CONGESTIVE OTITIS AS AN ISOLATED SYMPTOM OR THE INITIAL SYMPTOM OF AN INFECTIOUS DISEASE

The otalgia of inflammatory origin is isolated.

Oscillococcinum®

This is a remedy prepared from an aseptic filtered autolysate obtained from the liver and heart of the Muscovy duck (Anas barbariae). Its high **amino acid** content is probably the reason for the potentiation of the defense mechanisms of the organism against infectious agents.

Have the patient take a unit-dose tube as quickly as possible and repeat this dose three times every twenty-four hours.

Capsicum annuum

Experimentally, this substance causes and cures **hyperalgesic inflammation** in the **bones of the ear** with a **spreading** of the pain to the **mastoid** through localized congestive vasodilatation.

Prescribe five pellets in 5C every quarter of an hour, increasing the interval between doses as the pain is relieved.

Aconitum napellus

The indication of this remedy is motivated by the **appearance, especially at night**, of otalgia subsequent to the patient's exposure to a **sudden drop in temperature** (e.g. due to the north wind).

Either have the patient take a unit-dose tube of *Aconitum 9C*, one hour after a preliminary dose of *Oscillococcinum®*, or have him alternate a dose of five pellets of *Aconitum 9C* with a dose of five pellets of *Capsicum annuum 5C*, remembering to increase the interval between the doses as the intensity of the symptoms decreases.

Chamomilla

This remedy is prescribed for **children** or **hypersensitive people who cannot stand pain**. This definition applies perfectly to babies and young children during **teething**: they cry, they are agitated and can only be quieted down by being picked up or taken for a walk; inflammation of the ENT region accompanied by congestive otitis can also be observed during teething.

The symptoms are **exacerbated in the evening** between nine and midnight. The **cheek** on the side with the otitis is very often **hot and red**, while the other is cold and pale.

Prescribe five pellets of *Chamomilla 9* or *15C* (since there is a change in behavior) for each teething episode or agitation phase.

CONGESTIVE OTITIS AS A COMPLICATION OF RHINOPHARYNGITIS OR ADENOIDITIS

The otalgia progresses in the context of an acute febrile syndrome; in this case the following is used:

Oscillococcinum® in the same way as for isolated congestive otalgia.

Also, with regard to the intensity of the pain, *Capsicum annuum* and *Chamomilla* should be considered, as indicated above. To treat the acute febrile syndrome, use:

Aconitum napellus

Pathogenetic experimentation with *Aconitum* provokes shivering, then **marked hyperthermia** with a very rapid onset, **irritability of the heart, a warm, red, dry skin, intense thirst** (for cold water), **sthenic agitation,** and **otalgia**. This picture is often encountered after a sudden chill and often starts during the night (about midnight or one in the morning), waking the patient who then manifests a certain degree of anxiety.
Prescribe in medium dilution (9C), since there are both local and general symptoms, either one dose or doses of five pellets repeated every half-hour or every hour until the patient starts to sweat.

Belladonna

Pathogenetic experimentation with *Belladonna* provokes **intense, relapsing hyperthermia** with a very rapid onset, with irritability of the heart and **cephalic congestion** accompanied by throbbing pains, and a **red, radiantly warm** skin; the skin **on the face perspires profusely**.
Also noted are **intense thirst** because the mouth and the other mucous membranes are dry (sometimes dysphagia), photophobia due to mydriasis, **sensorial hyperesthesia** (to noise, touch, and jolts) and agitation with possible delirium or dejection.
The **eardrum** is quite **red**, the ear is sensitive to the least contact and the **pain is throbbing and nagging**.
Prescribe in medium dilutions (9C) if there are local and/or general symptoms in doses of five pellets approximately every hour, increasing the interval between doses as the intensity of the symptoms diminishes.
Prescribe in high dilutions (15 or 30C) if there are signs of nervous behavior as for example in the case of a child who is delirious or prone to febrile convulsions; prescribe doses of five pellets every 15 to 30 minutes, increasing the interval as the patient's condition improves.

Arsenicum album

The acute febrile syndrome sets in more or less rapidly; **the general state of the patient is affected** and alternates between **anxious agitation** and **dejection**. He experiences **intense thirst**. The otalgia takes the form of a **burning pain** which the patient automatically tries to relieve by applying **heat** locally, placing his hand or a cloth over the pinna of the ear; **nocturnal recrudescence** occurs between one and three in the morning.
Prescribe in repeated doses at 9C according to the nocturnal worsening of the symptoms.

Ferrum phosphoricum

The febrile syndrome is **more progressive at the onset**; the fever remains around 38.5° and is accompanied by a faster cardiac rhythm without irritability. The phenomena of vascular congestion can be seen in the face, which may be red or pale, in the nasal mucosa with possible epistaxis, the tracheal mucosa (dry cough), and the eardrum.
Since repeated doses of this medicine, especially in low dilutions, tends to incur quite frequently an aggravation of the acute congestion of the otitis, we prefer the administration of a single unit-dose tube of *Ferrum phosphoricum 9C* every twenty-four hours until the symptoms clear up.

2. SEROUS OTITIS

Serous otitis is a side effect of a rhinopharyngeal inflammation process spreading into the tympanic cavity via the eustachian tube. Since the lumen of the tube is physically obstructed

by inflammatory edema, the air in the tympanic cavity is not renewed entailing **hypersecretion of the epithelium of the cavity** with mucous or seromucous effusion.
The functional symptoms are much less obvious than in acute congestive otitis: the pain is rare and brief and sometimes there is none at all; the ear **feels blocked** (as with some cotton-wool) or **it feels full** and there is also **hypoacusis**; quite often the patients complain of buzzing and clicking noises when they swallow or blow their noses and also autophony (resonance of one's own voice when speaking).
Most of the time there are no general symptoms.
Examination reveals rhinopharyngitis in its final stage, and the otoscopy shows the **eardrum to be dull and retracted, of a bluish or yellowish gray**, sometimes covered with drops of serous fluid with the projection of the external apophysis of the hammer (because of rarefaction of the air). If the patient is examined standing up, **a certain level of liquid** is occasionally observed (presence of effusion).
To treat serous otitis, a choice should be made from the following:

Kali muriaticum

This remedy has a very particular affinity for the ENT region and allows effective treatment of coryza with blocked nostrils and catarrh in the eustachian tube.

To dry up the mucous secretion, prescribe *Kali muriaticum* in **at least 9C** in doses of five pellets three to four times during the day until the symptoms clear up.

Arsenicum iodatum

In spite of its limited proving, therapeutic experience has shown that this medicine is a very useful complement to the action of *Kali muriaticum*, especially in the case of an underlying allergic process. We therefore advise the alternate use of these two remedies; the dosage is the same.

Dulcamara

This medicine is indicated for catarrh in the ENT region with a sensation of blocked nose and ears and possibly a cough and hoarseness. Although it is more particularly a remedy for chronic diseases, the prescription of this substance belongs in this chapter if the etiology highlights the notions of **cold and humidity** (serous otitis occurring after the patient has gotten wet, in rainy or foggy weather).

Prescribe in 9C once or twice a day until the symptoms clear up.

Manganum aceticum

This medicine is typically confused with *Manganum metallicum* although the proving was carried out using manganese acetate; it is indicated for tubal catarrh **preceded or accompanied by hoarseness**.

Prescribe in 9C once or twice a day.

Mercurius dulcis

Although often cited, this medicine has always seemed to us to be consistently ineffective.

• • • • • • • • •

Thus treated (essentially using *Kali muriaticum*, *Arsenicum iodatum*, and *Dulcamara*), serous otitis can be satisfactorily cured in five or six days, without risk of progression towards superinfection or an adhesive scar.

3. SUPPURATIVE OTITIS

Suppurative otitis corresponds to a **purulent collection** on the inside of the eardrum causing very painful high pressure in the tympanic cavity. If the pressure is too great the eardrum is quickly perforated; this perforation may be sufficiently large and allow the discharge of the pus into the external acoustic meatus, thus bringing almost instant relief from the pain with rapid regression of the general signs. But the perforation may only let a few drops of pus seep out and then the regression of the pain and of the general signs is only temporary.

When the patient is seen for the first time during this stage and the pus cannot be discharged conveniently in a spontaneous manner, it is essential to drain the pus, i.e. carry out **paracentesis**. In this case, the homeopathic treatment becomes the therapeutic complement of this operation, helping the infection to clear up.

The general signs consist of **very intense pain, fever** and a change in behavior (**agitation, prostration**, or both alternately) which in most cases progress in parallel until there is a build-up of pus on the inside of the eardrum: these signs diminish with the discharge of the pus.

When examining the patient, the eardrum appears **pinkish-gray with a bulge** in the upper posterior quarter if the purulent collection is retained; the external acoustic meatus is flooded with creamy, yellowish pus with sometimes a nauseating smell if there is a fistula.

While waiting for paracentesis,

Lachesis mutus

is the most preferred medicine as the use of this venom is justified by the modality of **aggravation** of the symptoms in the **absence** or **cessation of the discharge** of the pathologic secretion. The left lateral dominance which is characteristic of the proving of this medicine is ignored for the choice of remedy.

Prescribe a unit-dose tube of *Lachesis 9* or *15C*.

When the draining has been correctly accomplished, a choice should be made from among the following remedies:

Pyrogenium

This nosode is prepared from a septic autolysate of beef, pork, and human placenta; it may be **systematically** prescribed for any painful suppurative phenomenon which is improved by the local application of heat, especially if there is a concomitant febrile reaction.

Prescribe five pellets a day or a daily unit-dose tube of *Pyrogenium 9C* for between five and seven days, in addition to the symptomatic homeopathic medicines.

Hepar sulphur

This medicine complements *Pyrogenium* in acute suppurative processes (see the chapter entitled "Abscesses and Acute Suppurative Processes", p. 93). Low dilutions which encourage suppuration should be avoided.

The prescription of four doses "in scaled dosage" provides a maximum of safety and results: it involves prescribing a daily dose of *Hepar sulphur* in increasing dilutions over four consecutive days: 9C the first day, 12C the second day, 15C the third day, and 30C the fourth day. Each dose is preceded two hours earlier by a dose of *Pyrogenium 9C.*

Aviaire

The tuberculin of birds, which is obtained from antiseptic-free cultures of Mycobacterium tuberculosis of avian origin, has a more specific action on the ear than *Tuberculinum*; it is appropriate for weak and anorexic people, notably children in whom the slightest rhinopharyngitis degenerates into ENT or bronchial complications. It has the advantage of being able to be used during the course, or at the abating, of acute or subacute otitis.
This remedy is therefore indicated in the acute or subacute period in children presenting **recurring otitis**. A single dose in 15C improves the current symptoms and is the first stage in a constitutional treatment.

Kali bichromicum

Often associated with a greenish-yellow mucopurulent form of rhinorrhea which is stringy, viscous, and sticky, the otorrhea requiring *Kali bichromicum* is **more mucous than purulent**, stretching into **long filaments,** and sometimes giving off a fetid smell.

Prescribe five pellets two to four times a day in at least 9C to help check the otorrhea.

Hydrastis canadensis

Frequently accompanied by very thick and viscous rhinorrhea, the otorrhea requiring *Hydrastis* is **purulent, viscous, and greenish-yellow**, with no fetid smell.

Same dosage as for *Kali bichromicum.*

Mercurius solubilis

The otorrhea is **profuse, mucopurulent, greenish-yellow, caustic** for the external acoustic meatus and gives off a **bad smell**.

The patient is febrile and sweats with shivers on the surface of the skin; an increase in sialorrhea and a limp, flaccid tongue with tooth marks can also be observed.

Same dosage.

Arsenicum album

This medicine is indicated for purulent otorrhea with a discharge which is **quite fluid, beige**, obviously **excoriating** on the external acoustic meatus, and has a **repulsive smell**. Also, the **general state** of the patient is **changed**, since he shows a **high fever**, with alternating periods of **anxious agitation and dejection**, and **intense thirst**. The symptoms are aggravated at night and improved by local heat.

N.B.: An acute febrile gastroenteritic syndrome may be associated with the complaint and may even be the reason for the consultation if the patient is a baby.

Same dosage as for the previous remedies.

Aurum muriaticum

For the reasons given on p. 96, this remedy rather than *Aurum metallicum* is indicated for suppuration in small bones in general and, in particular, suppurative processes in the vicinity of the auditory ossicles.

Prescribe five pellets once a day in at least 9C.

EXAMPLES OF PRESCRIPTIONS

1ST EXAMPLE

Take the case of a child with acute non-febrile otalgia occurring a few hours after a winter sports class with the north wind blowing. On examination, the eardrum is congested and pinkish and there are no other symptoms.

Prescription

1. Take as quickly as possible a unit-dose tube of
   Oscillococcinum®

and repeat this dose every morning for the next three days.

2. Every quarter of an hour take alternate doses of five pellets of
   Aconitum 9C (1 multi-dose tube)
   and five pellets of
   Capsicum annuum 5C (1 multi-dose tube).

Increase the interval between doses as the intensity of the symptoms diminishes.

2ND EXAMPLE

Take the case of a teenager who consults the practitioner for reduced auditory acuity which he has had for a few days. On examination, the eardrum is dull, bluish and it is revealed that the patient tried out a wind-surfing board for the first time ten days before. Valsalva's maneuver produces a clicking sound in the ear.

Prescription

1. On awakening and at bedtime take five pellets of
   Dulcamara 9C (1 multi-dose tube).
2. Approximately every two hours during the day, the patient should take alternatively a dose of five pellets of
   Kali muriaticum 9C (2 multi-dose tubes)
   and a dose of five pellets of
   Arsenicum iodatum 9C (2 multi-dose tubes).

Increase the interval between doses as the intensity of the symptoms diminishes.

3RD EXAMPLE

Take the case of a child who a few days before had shown signs of excoriating acute rhinopharyngitis, quickly turning greenish, with profuse, burning lacrimation. The previous night, his temperature went up to 40°C, and he was agitated at different times in the night, being woken by very painful otalgia. He kept putting his hand over his ear and asked several times for a drink of cold water. In the morning his parents noticed a purulent discharge in his ear.

On examination, the child is febrile with a temperature of 38.7°C; greenish rhinitis with excoriation of the nostrils is noted, his throat is inflamed and his mouth is full of saliva. The otorrhea is greenish, seeping into the whole of the external acoustic meatus and giving off a repulsive smell.

Prescription

1. For four consecutive mornings, prescribe a unit-dose tube of
   Pyrogenium 9C (4 doses)

followed two hours later by a unit-dose tube of
Hepar sulphur 9C on the first day,
Hepar sulphur 12C on the second day,
Hepar sulphur 15C on the third day,
Hepar sulphur 30C on the fourth day.

2. During the day, take alternate doses every hour of five pellets of

   Arsenicum album 9C (2 multi-dose tubes)

   and five pellets of

   Mercurius solubilis 9C (2 multi-dose tubes).

Increase the interval between doses as the intensity of the symptoms diminishes.

•••••••••

HOARSENESS AND APHONIA

Hoarseness consists of a change in the voice and **aphonia** a loss of voice.

These forms of **dysphonia** originate from trouble in the larynx whose origin will possibly have to be identified by:

- an examination of the larynx to find a local cause: infection, inflammation, neoplastic tumor, polyp, compression, paralysis;
- a general examination: nervous cause, hysteria, etc.

Homeopathy is effective:

- in cases of hoarseness and aphonia resulting from overexertion of the voice, or in cases of dysphonia in the asthenic patient;
- for hoarseness or aphonia of non-specific infectious origin of recent date. Since in such cases it is mostly a question of viral origin, prescribe a dose of *Oscillococcinum*® as soon as possible, to be repeated six hours later since clinical practice has proved the effectiveness of this remedy at the onset of viral complaints (see the chapter entitled "Acute Laryngitis and Tracheitis" for the complementary symptomatic remedies).

We shall only deal here with remedies for overexertion of the voice and dysphonia in asthenic patients.

HOARSENESS DUE TO OVEREXERTION OF THE VOICE

Arum triphyllum

This remedy is indicated for cases of hoarseness with a **double tonal voice**: the timbre of the voice varies constantly; it is sometimes clear, sometimes husky, depending on the tone.

Prescribe five pellets in 5C every two hours increasing the interval between doses as the condition improves.

Rhus toxicodendron

This remedy is indicated for hoarseness with the characteristic modality of the proving: **improvement with moving**.

The hoarseness appears only at the beginning of the speech or the song, then improves progressively to reappear, however, when the patient is tired.

Prescribe *Rhus toxicodendron* in 9C, five pellets once or twice in the hour preceding the use of the voice.

Arnica

Indicated when the hoarseness is the **result of excessive fatigue in the vocal cords**: aphonia after speaking too much, shouting too much, singing too much, etc.

Prescribe five pellets in 9C two to four times a day.

Argentum metallicum

Indicated in particular for **pharyngitis in singers or speakers**: hoarseness or aphonia with the sensation of an open wound in the larynx. Aggravation when coughing, swallowing, or speaking. The cough may produce thick, grayish, viscous mucus.

Argentum nitricum

This remedy is preferred if the patient **feels a splinter-like pain in the throat**, with a constant urge to "clear his throat". The *Argentum nitricum* type of hoarseness may also have emotional causes, e.g. nervous apprehension.

Prescribe in 5C, five pellets every two hours. Increase interval with improvement.

Manganum aceticum

This remedy is more specifically suited to cases of hoarseness brought on by humid cold or prolonged speaking.

Sensation of stinging in the larynx spreading to the ears.

Left untreated these types of hoarseness are frequently complicated by bronchitis.

Prescribe in 5C, two to four times a day. Increase interval with improvement.

Causticum

This medicine is indicated for **paralysis of the vocal cords** after intense use of the voice or after viral infections.

The hoarseness is **worse in the morning, when the larynx feels raw**. It is **improved by taking a drink of cold water**.

Prescribe in 5C, five pellets two to four times a day depending on the seriousness of the case. Increase interval with improvement.

Phosphorus

This remedy is to be prescribed for hoarseness which is **aggravated in the evening** and in the first part of the night. The larynx is very painful and the patient is unable to speak because of the pain.

Same dosage as for *Causticum*.

Magnesia carbonica and Graphites

These two remedies are indicated for women who have sore throats with **aphonia before** (*Magnesia carbonica*) and **during** (*Graphites*) **periods**.

Prescribe five pellets in 7C twice a day, a few days before the time the problems usually occur.

DYSPHONIA IN ASTHENIC PATIENTS

These cases involve functional dysphonia in asthenic patients arising from physical reasons or caused by emotional overload. The anxiety provokes muscular tension and an incorrect use of the air stream in these patients.

The practitioner should therefore prescribe, in addition to one of the preceding medicines, a remedy which corresponds to the global reactive mode of these patients until the fatigue or the anxiety improves.

Phosphoricum acidum

Indicated in asthenic individuals after **emotional shocks** or **overwork**.

Prescribe in 15C, once or twice weekly.

Kali phosphoricum

Indicated in asthenic individuals when there is also **nervous irritability** after overwork.

Prescribe in 9C, once a day.

Ignatia

Indicated when there is **extreme irritability and hyperesthesia of all the senses** with the sensation of a ball in the throat and a need to give a sigh. The symptomatology is accompanied by **paradoxical modalities**.

Prescribe in 9C, five pellets every morning on awakening.

•••••••••

ACUTE TONSILLITIS

Tonsillitis is an acute or subacute inflammation of the oropharynx which may affect both tonsils, or only one of them, spread to the uvula, the pillars, the soft palate, and the posterior wall of the pharynx.

Homeopathic therapy is effective in most cases in dealing with these complaints which may provide an opening for remote infections (acute articular rheumatism, nephritis, etc.). If the practitioner, however, is unsure of the reactive potential of a patient affected with tonsillitis caused by group A streptococci, treatment with antibiotics may perfectly well be combined with the remedies indicated by the patient's symptoms.

Clinically, the following can be distinguished:

- **erythematous tonsillitis**;
- **erythematous pharyngitis and laryngopharyngitis with false membrane**;
- **necrotic ulcerating pharyngitis** (presence of one or more ulcerations);
- **phlegmonous pharyngitis**.

Each of these clinical forms presents local signs and general signs to which some of the provings of our remedies correspond.

Excluded from this study are diphtherial tonsillitis and necrotic ulcerating pharyngitis which is symptomatic of malignant hemopathy.

ERYTHEMATOUS TONSILLITIS

There are three prime remedies worthy of note:

Belladonna

Local symptoms

The mucous membrane of the throat is **red, dry, and painful when swallowing**. Occasionally a **spasmodic contraction** of the throat muscles makes the patient feel that a hand is squeezing his throat. This sensation is aggravated when swallowing and the **pain may spread towards the ears**. Quite often the cervical ganglions are swollen and painful.

General symptoms

The patient has a **high, fluctuant temperature. His head** feels **congested and he sweats profusely**. The general modalities of the remedy can be observed:

aggravation due to light, noise, contact, and cold air; improvement in darkness and quiet.

Prescribe in 5 or 9C, five pellets every two or three hours. Increase interval with improvement.

Apis mellifica

Local symptoms

The pharyngeal mucous membrane and the tonsils are **edematous** and **red pink**. The uvula hangs like a bag full of water. The **pains** are **stinging and burning, improved by drinking cold water** or sucking ice.

General symptoms

There is a high fever. The skin is alternately dry and sweating. **The patient is not thirsty**.

Prescribe five pellets in 9C every hour. *Apis* has a rapid though short-lasting action. Increase interval with improvement.

Phytolacca decandra

Local symptoms

The pharynx is **dark red, notably on the pillars of the soft palate**. The tonsils are swollen and the uvula is sometimes edematous, but less so than with *Apis*. Swallowing causes a pain **which spreads into the ears**. There are sometimes little white dots which make up a false membrane and give the impression of a foreign body in the mouth and a constant need to swallow. The **cervical ganglions** are **inflamed and hypertrophied**.

General symptoms

These are less obvious than the symptoms of the preceding remedies; there may be myalgia or the body may feel as if it is bruised all over.

Prescribe in 5C, five pellets every two or three hours, sometimes alternately with *Belladonna*.

ERYTHEMATOUS PHARYNGITIS AND LARYNGOPHARYNGITIS WITH FALSE MEMBRANE

Four mercury salts are especially homeopathic to this type of pharyngitis:

Mercurius solubilis

Local symptoms

The pharynx and the tonsils are red with dysphagia spreading to the ears; there are little white dots or thick false membranes present. **The tongue has a characteristic aspect**: flabby and enlarged with tooth marks along the sides. It is covered with a **thick yellowish coating**. **The breath is fetid**, the saliva profuse and thick. **Presence of cervical adenopathy**.

General symptoms

The patient's fever is high and constant. He is given to shivering on the surface of the skin and profuse sweating which affords no relief. Intense thirst.

Dosage

Low dilutions (5C) tend to promote suppuration. Therefore, the remedy should be more readily prescribed in 9C, five pellets every two or three hours, or else in 15C in patients subject to phlegmon.

The taking of this medicine alternately with *Belladonna* covers the reactive modalities in more than 80% of the cases of tonsillitis: the large majority of patients with tonsillitis, in fact, show simultaneously or alternately similar symptoms to those which are caused by these two substances in the healthy person. Rummel, a disciple of Hahnemann, first noticed this in 1849.

Mercurius bi-iodatus and proto-iodatus

Local symptoms

These relate to one-sided or predominantly one-sided erythematous or pultaceous tonsillitis. *Mercurius bi-iodatus* is indicated for complaints which have an affinity for the left tonsil and *Mercurius proto-iodatus* for those which target the right tonsil.

General symptoms

These are the same as for *Mercurius solubilis.*

Prescribe one dose in 9C of the chosen salt, morning and evening.

....

EXAMPLE OF PRESCRIPTION FOR A RIGHT-SIDED ERYTHEMATOUS PHARYNGITIS

- Take a unit-dose tube morning and evening of
  Mercurius proto-iodatus 9C (six doses).

- During the day, take alternate doses approximately every two hours of five pellets of
  Belladonna 9C (one tube),

and five pellets of
  Mercurius solubilis 9C (one tube).

Increase the interval between doses as the patient's condition improves.

Mercurius cyanatus

Local symptoms

The pharynx has **grayish, sticky false membranes**, covering bleeding ulcerations, which are difficult to detach. The **cervical adenopathy** is **painful** to touch.

General symptoms

The patient's overall condition is affected and there is also prostration.

Homeopaths used to consider *Mercurius cyanatus* "the" remedy for diphtherial tonsillitis. It can still be an effective adjuvant to the serotherapy of this complaint.

For serious non-diphtherial laryngopharyngitis with false membrane, prescribe one unit-dose tube of *Mercurius cyanatus* morning and evening. During the day, take alternate doses every two hours of five pellets of *Belladonna 9C* and five pellets of *Mercurius solubilis* or *Mercurius corrosivus 9C,* depending on the clinical symptoms.

MALIGNANT AND NECROTIC ULCERATING PHARYNGITIS

Mercurius corrosivus

Local symptoms

This remedy is suitable for **throat ulcers** which spread rapidly, **burning like hot embers**, on a swollen, painful, inflamed mucous membrane. The pain is aggravated by the slightest contact. **Swallowing is hyperalgesic**, even in the case of liquids; it causes **spasms and constriction** in the throat. The ganglions in the neck are hypertrophied and hypersensitive.

General symptoms

These are the same as for *Mercurius solubilis.*

Prescribe five pellets in9C four times a day.

Lachesis mutus

Local symptoms

The tonsils are swollen, ulcerated and are a **dark red color**; they produce a constrictive sensation and **the slightest exterior contact is not tolerated. Swallowing saliva and hot liquids is more difficult than swallowing solids and cold liquids**.

General symptoms

The patient's overall condition is seriously affected, with dejection and adynamia.

Prescribe in 9 or 15C, five pellets twice a day.

Kali bichromicum

Local symptoms

These are mostly **regularly-edged ulcers** with **adhesive, yellow or greenish-yellow viscous exudation**. They are especially found on the pillars of the soft palate; they cause localized edema on the uvula which makes it hang like a little bag full of water (*Apis*).

General symptoms

These are rather discreet.

Prescribe in 5C, five pellets two to four times a day depending on the seriousness of the case.

Ailanthus glandulosa

Local symptoms

The throat is dark red with little purplish spots or ulcers. The tongue is dry and sometimes brown, and **swallowing is very painful**. There is **very extensive and sensitive cervical adenopathy**. The breath is fetid.

General symptoms

The general condition is markedly affected: **adynamia**, **prostration**, and **stupor** with the face congested and bloated.

This remedy is indicated for **monocytic** tonsillitis or for some malignant types of tonsillitis, and may be combined with conventional treatments if necessary.

Prescribe five pellets in 5C every six hours approximately.

Arum triphyllum

Local symptoms

The pharynx is **bright red**. There is sharp, stricture-type pain. **The saliva is profuse. The tongue** may be **raspberry-colored**, and clear of papillae.

General symptoms

These are **severe**: the temperature is very high. The patient may be prostrate or agitated. **He is constantly tearing little scales from his lips** with his fingers or teeth with **occasional bleeding**.

This is therefore a remedy for serious cases of tonsillitis, often related to scarlet fever. Nowadays it is essentially used as a support for treatment with antibiotics.

Prescribe five pellets in 5C four times per day.

PHLEGMONOUS PHARYNGITIS

The homeopathic treatment **should be prescribed early on**. Otherwise the treatment will be essentially with antibiotics or surgical.

Pyrogenium

This nosode is a remedy which should be used for all serious infections in which the general condition is affected and pulse and temperature are dissociated. The secretions have a putrid smell. It is not necessary, nor desirable, to wait for this clinical stage to prescribe the remedy since it is very reliable for preventing or stopping suppurative processes. It should be used right at the beginning before the purulent collection forms, or, conversely, when the suppuration is in the process of draining. It should be avoided when the purulent mass has collected since it would then delay the maturation of the abscess and the evacuation of the pus.

Prescribe a unit-dose tube in 9C in association with:

Hepar sulphur

This is the fundamental remedy for acute suppuration. The dosage obeys very strict rules related to the differences in the remedy's action which varies with the dilution:

- **high dilutions** (15-30C) **check** or resorb the suppuration;
- **low dilutions** (5C) **favor** suppuration;
- **medium dilutions** (9C) **might be ambivalent** and act in one way or the other depending on the clinical stage of the suppuration.

At the onset of a phlegmon of the tonsil, it is effective to use the so-called "scaled" method of prescription:

- at the onset of the infection, take a tube of *Pyrogenium 9C* and, two hours later, a unit-dose tube of *Hepar sulphur 9C;*
- twelve hours later, take a unit-dose tube of *Hepar sulphur 12C,* still preceded two hours earlier by a unit-dose tube of *Pyrogenium 9C;*
- twenty-four hours later, a unit-dose tube of *Hepar sulphur 15C,* preceded two hours earlier by a dose of *Pyrogenium 9C;*
- twenty-four hours later, a unit-dose tube of *Hepar sulphur 30C,* again two hours after a unit-dose tube of *Pyrogenium 9C.*

●●●●●●●●●

In all cases of tonsillitis it is very useful to prescribe gargling with 20 drops of a mixture of equal parts of *Phytolacca MT* and *Calendula MT* in a glass of lukewarm water four to five times a day, in addition to the general treatment. This local treatment has a remarkable antalgic and antiseptic power.

●●●●●●●●●

ACUTE LARYNGITIS AND TRACHEITIS

Acute laryngitis and tracheitis are bouts of dry coughing of rapid onset; they may be isolated cases or the start of an infectious, possibly febrile, episode and are due to an inflammatory reaction in the upper air passages. Some forms are of dystonic origin.

The homeopathic medicines are selected from those whose provings correspond to the first, inflammatory, stage. We shall distinguish the following in our presentation:

- laryngotracheitis appearing at the onset of a febrile syndrome,
- laryngitis stridulosa,
- tussigenic laryngitis,
- laryngitis with dysphonia,
- acute tracheitis,
- spasmodic tracheitis caused by neurovegetative dystonia.

CONCOMITANT LARYNGOTRACHEITIS AT THE ONSET OF A FEBRILE SYNDROME

The cough and fever appear almost simultaneously.

Aconitum napellus

Pathogenetic experimentation with *Aconitum* provokes, after a shiver, **intense hyperthermia** with very rapid onset, accompanied by **irritability of the heart, a red, warm skin which is dry, intense thirst** (for cold water) and **sthenic agitation**. Simultaneously, there is a **hoarse, dry, croupy cough**. This picture is often encountered after a sudden chill and is liable to begin at night-time (about midnight or one in the morning) waking the patient who then appears to be quite anxious; concomitant otalgia may be observed.

Prescribe the medicine in medium dilutions (9C) since there are simultaneously local and general symptoms, in doses of five pellets to be repeated every half-hour or every hour until sweating begins which indicates that *Aconitum* should be replaced by *Belladonna*. If the cough shows one of the characteristic modalities described in the study of the homeopathic medicines for acute laryngitis and tracheitis, then alternate *Aconitum* with the suitably chosen symptomatic medicine.

Belladonna

The proving of this remedy causes relapsing **hyperthermia** with a very rapid onset, accompanied by **irritability of the heart** and **cephalic congestion** with throbbing pains, **a red and radiantly warm skin which perspires, especially in the face**; dryness in the mucous membranes which produces **intense thirst, a short, dry cough**, a tickling in the throat, and dysphagia are also noted. There is also **photophobia** due to mydriasis, sensory hyperesthesia (to noise, touch, jolts), and agitation with the possibility of delirium or dejection.

Prescribe the medicine in medium dilution (9C), if not in high dilution (15C), for a child who is delirious or prone to febrile convulsions, in doses of five pellets repeated every half-hour or every hour approximately with progressively greater intervals as the intensity of the symptoms decreases.

LARYNGITIS STRIDULOSA

Laryngitis stridulosa is an attack of acute dyspnea with sudden onset which is due to a sudden inflammation of the larynx and is accompanied by a striking dry, hoarse, barking cough that impresses the patient and his family. The fit may be isolated or it may be the beginning of a rhinopharyngeal infectious episode; it may or may not be febrile. Improvement comes with any form of heat: wrapping up well around the neck, inhalation of hot water vapors, and hot drinks. Finally, it is practically only observed in young children with hypertrophy of the adenoid vegetation, or in nervous children.

The homeopathic medicines are selected from those whose provings correspond to the first stage of the inflammation, and which display an affinity for the larynx and improvement with heat. In this way, a rapid remission is effected and respiratory distress, a complication which is always possible, is avoided.

Spongia tosta

This remedy is indicated for a **dry**, croupy, wheezing **cough like the noise of a saw cutting through a pine plank**, or a dog coughing. The nasal and pharyngeal mucous membranes are dry; there is a **burning**, **suffocating** sensation of stricture provoking much anxiety. Improvement is observed after **drinking something hot**.

Prescribe in 5C, five pellets every five to ten minutes, alternating, as required, doses of *Aconitum* or *Belladonna* if there is an associated fever with corresponding modalities. Increase the interval between doses progressively as the intensity of the symptoms decreases.

Sambucus nigra

This medicine is prescribed for a **sudden sensation of suffocation** with **wheezing inspiration** about midnight, with the expiration hindered by **thick mucus** which is difficult to shift, and nasal obstruction. The patient displays **profuse sweating** in the face on awakening; he is unable to keep his head down and sits up in bed, showing increasing signs of **cyanosis**. Improvement is observed following the application of **hot compresses** to the front of the neck. Check that it is not a case of epiglottiditis requiring a tracheal operation.

Same dosage as for *Spongia tosta*.

Hepar sulphur

This remedy is used when the laryngitis stridulosa is accompanied by **intense pain** in the throat (as if there was a fish bone stuck) making the patient **irritable**. Improvement is effected by inhaling **hot humid air** and applying **hot compresses**. These signs are most frequently observed in difficult children who show a tendency towards suppuration after a sudden chill.

Prescribe the medicine in a single dose at the start of the treatment in high dilution (15 or 30C) because of the continuous risk of possible underlying purulent otitis; then prescribe the suitable remedy or remedies.

TUSSIGENIC LARYNGITIS

Although responsible for coughing fits, the inflammation of the larynx is less intensive than in laryngitis stridulosa; there is only a permanent tickling in the larynx or short laryngeal spasms provoking coughing bouts.

Coccus cacti

A **tickling in the larynx** is the cause of a fitful cough entailing the **expectoration of stringy**, viscous **mucus**, **especially on awakening** and in the evening **about eleven**. The cough is relieved by cool air or a drink of cold water.

Prescribe in 5C to be taken before the usual time of the coughing bouts.

Cuprum metallicum

This is for a dry, **pertussoid**, **spasmodic cough**, with suffocation and cyanosis due to a laryngeal spasm occurring during the fits which are **relieved by drinking cold water**. A pseudo-convulsive aspect with spasms throughout the whole body can sometimes be observed in children, as well as the child's thumb folded into the clenched fist.

Prescribe *Cuprum 9C* in doses of five pellets to be taken when there is a coughing fit. *Cuprum oxydatum* is to be preferred to *Cuprum metallicum* when the cough is concomitant with oxyuriasis.

Mephitis putorius

Occurring approximately **every two hours**, a laryngeal spasm blocks expiration, thus provoking a reflex, spasmodic cough and cyanosis in the face.

Prescribe five pellets of *Mephitis putorius 5C* to be taken with each fit of coughing.

LARYNGITIS WITH DYSPHONIA

Arum triphyllum

There is intense inflammation with marked dryness in the lips, nasopharynx and larynx.

Hoarseness and a **bitonal voice** are heard; the cough is husky. According to the usual description, the patient chews or scratches his lips until they bleed.

Prescribe five pellets in 5C every hour, steadily increasing the interval between doses.

Ammonium causticum

This remedy is prescribed for a **continuous, suffocating cough**, with **hoarseness** and the sensation that the **mucous membrane** in the larynx is **raw**.

Prescribe in 5C every hour. Increase interval with improvement.

ACUTE TRACHEITIS

Acute tracheitis is an inflammation of the trachea due to microbial agents which produces a pathologic picture limited to bouts of dry, exhausting coughing which may or may not be febrile. The spontaneous progression may be downwards, veering towards acute bronchitis (see the chapter devoted to this subject, p. 152).

FEBRILE ACUTE TRACHEITIS

There are of course *Aconitum* and *Belladonna* for a sudden febrile invasion.

Bryonia

The febrile condition has a **progressive onset** and the dryness of the mucous membranes causes **intense thirst**. The **cough** is **dry** and is provoked or **aggravated by the slightest movement**, or by speaking or entering a warm bedroom. This cough is painful, causing sternal and thoracic pain whose intensity is reduced by applying pressure to the thorax with the hands.

Prescribe *Bryonia 9C*, in doses of five pellets approximately every two hours or in time with the coughing fits. Increase interval with improvement. Combine it on occasion with *Ferrum phosphoricum*.

NON-FEBRILE ACUTE TRACHEITIS

Drosera

The cough is dry and spasmodic, **especially in nocturnal bouts** when the patient is lying down. The respiration is wheezy and cyanosis in the face can be observed. Costal or abdominal pain is improved by the pressure of the hands.

Since low dilutions risk causing aggravation, prescribe *Drosera* in at least 9C, in doses of five pellets, if not a unit-dose tube in 30C at bedtime.

Sticta pulmonaria

The cough is dry, irritant, continuous and tiring, with **dryness of the nasal mucous membrane**. There is a sensation of obstruction at the bridge of the nose and of heaviness as if the nose were being pinched by a pince-nez, and also a constant need to blow the nose without result.

Prescribe in 5C, five pellets every hour, often alternating with *Bryonia* which it complements favorably.

Rumex crispus

This medicine is indicated for an **itch in the substernal fossa** provoking a continual, reflex dry cough, **aggravated by breathing in cold air** to the extent that the patient has to breathe through a handkerchief or a cloth wrapped around the nose and mouth.

Prescribe in 5C to be taken with the coughing bout.

Corallium rubrum

The cough is violent, spasmodic, **explosive**, uncontrollable, accompanied by the **vomiting of stringy mucus** causing **redness in the face**; the pharynx is red. The patient covers his head with the blankets **to avoid breathing cool air** which seems to provoke the coughing fits.

Prescribe in 5C at the same rate as the fits of coughing.

SPASMODIC TRACHEITIS DUE TO NEUROVEGETATIVE DYSTONIA

The cough appears in hypersensitive people in a particular context.

Ignatia amara

The more the patient coughs, the more he wants to cough; he describes the impression of having a lump in his throat.

The **modalities** of the cough are always **paradoxical**: for example, the cough is set off by other people's smoke but if the patient himself smokes, he does not cough.

Prescribe five pellets of *Ignatia* 9C once or twice a day.

Hyoscyamus niger

This involves a nocturnal coughing fit, **appearing as soon as the patient lies down** and stopping when he sits up.

Prescribe in 9C, five pellets before bedtime.

ACUTE BRONCHITIS

Acute bronchitis is a local or wider inflammation of the bronchi. The most usual cause is infectious, whether viral or bacterial.

No anomaly shows up on an X-ray. When anomalies do appear it is because the inflammation has affected the pulmonary alveoli.

Clinically, acute bronchitis shows itself as a more or less intense febrile syndrome, accompanied by a cough.

The progression of the disease may produce a lot of complications in the elderly patient and the patient suffering from a heart condition or chronic respiratory insufficiency.

In children, acute bronchitis is often concomitant with or consequent to ENT infections and may sometimes be accompanied by pulmonary complaints.

The homeopathic remedies chosen differ according to whether the patient is seen at the onset stage, the fully-declared phase, or the resolution phase.

PERIOD OF ONSET

There is a febrile condition with a dry, non-productive cough.

Aconitum napellus

Intense hyperthermia with a sudden onset appears after a **sudden chill**. The skin is red and **dry**. The patient shows **intense thirst** for large quantities of cold water.

The **cough is dry and painful**. Although generally **sthenic and vigorous**, the patient may be agitated, if not anxious.

Prescribe five pellets every hour in 9C. The indication for this remedy is short-lived for this first stage of the inflammation; it ceases as soon as sweating begins, to be replaced by:

Belladonna

This remedy corresponds to the following clinical picture: hyperthermia with sudden onset with

extensive cephalic congestion. The face is red and **sweating profuse**. The patient is dejected but **hyperesthetic** to noise, light, and jolts and often has a throbbing headache.

The **fever may fluctuate**. **The cough is dry, spasmodic**, and painful with dryness in the throat.

Prescribe in 9C, five pellets every two hours. Increase interval with improvement.

During this onset period, the dry, unproductive cough will be improved, depending on its specific modalities, by:

Rumex crispus

For a dry, tiring cough provoked by an itching in the substernal recess, with the impression of a **tickling in the recess** and sometimes a sensation of a grazed throat. The cough is **aggravated by breathing cool air,** when going from the heat into the cold, in proportion to the volume of air breathed in, and relieved by closing the mouth or **covering the nose and mouth**.

Prescribe *Rumex 5C*, five pellets to be taken with the fits of coughing.

Sticta pulmonaria

A spasmodic, dry cough with the sensation of a burning graze in the trachea. Aggravation at night or in a cold bedroom. Improvement on sitting up.

At the same time as the cough, there may sometimes be redness in the cheeks but especially **a dry nasal mucous membrane with the impression that the nose is blocked at the bridge** which is the site of a pinching pain "like wearing tightly-fitted glasses".

Prescribe *Sticta 5C*, five pellets every two or three hours depending on the seriousness of the case. Increase interval with improvement.

Bryonia

Febrile state with **progressive onset**. A dry cough, **provoked or aggravated by the slightest movement**, even respiratory movement. The patient tries to remain immobile. He is intensely **thirsty**. He sweats profusely, which brings relief.

Prescribe five pellets in 9C three to four times per day. Increase interval with improvement.

Drosera

A spasmodic, dry cough appearing in fits, **especially at night** when lying down, and sometimes cyanosis in the face and wheezing respiration. Associated costal or abdominal pains, relieved by the pressure of the hands.

Prescribe in 15 or 30C, once a day until the cough clears up. It seemed to us that low or medium dilutions might cause aggravation.

FULLY-DECLARED PHASE

At this stage the cough becomes productive, bringing mucous or mucopurulent expectoration.

Ferrum phosphoricum

The temperature is not very high in a weak, hyposthenic **person**. The patient readily presents congestion and pallor in the face alternately and is subject to **epistaxis**. The spasmodic cough, initially dry, is very **painful**, with a **burning sensation in the chest**. Aggravation in the cold air or lying down. Then there is a small amount of yellow expectoration which is sometimes streaked with blood.

Prescribe five pellets in 9C, three or four times per day. Increase interval with improvement.

Ipeca

The cough is spasmodic and is **accompanied by nausea and vomiting**. It is aggravated by movement, improved by rest, and may be accompanied by **epistaxis**. There is an accumulation of mucus in the bronchi with disseminated rale (gurgling and/or sibilant rale), but **little expectoration**. In these conditions, the **emetic cough** may become **dyspneic or asthmatic**.

In spite of the associated digestive symptoms, the tongue is clear or lightly coated. The nausea is accompanied **by hypersalivation with absence of thirst**.

Prescribe in 9C, five pellets in time with the coughing fits.

Mercurius solubilis

A productive, loose cough with **mucopurulent expectoration**, aggravated at night in the warmth of the bed. The patient presents shivering on the surface of the skin. There are **concomitant, buccopharyngeal signs**: the tongue is wide, flabby, thick, and sprawling; it retains the marks of the teeth along the sides and is covered with a thick, yellowish coating. Fetid breath, **hypersalivation, intense thirst** (the *Ipeca* patient also has hypersalivation, but the tongue is clear or lightly coated, with absence of thirst).

Prescribe five pellets in 9C twice a day.

Hepar sulphur

With this remedy, the cough is first of all dry; then there is suppuration with **profuse purulent expectoration** and moist rale.

Dosage

The action of *Hepar sulphur* in dealing with suppuration depends on the strength of the dilution used:

- **The low dilutions** (5C) **enhance suppuration** and play a centrifugal role (as for low dilutions of *Sulphur*, there is a possible aggravation of suppuration in an enclosed cavity, e.g. otitis). *Hepar sulphur* in 5C favors expectoration at the onset. Prescribe five pellets twice a day.
- **The high dilutions** (15-30C) **check suppuration**. *Hepar sulphur 15C* dries up expectoration. Prescribe five pellets once or twice a day.

The technique of "scaled dosage" can also be used; it consists in prescribing:

Hepar sulphur 9C, one dose on the first day,

Hepar sulphur 12C, one dose on the second day,

Hepar sulphur 15C, one dose on the third day,

Hepar sulphur 30C, one dose on the fourth day.

Each dose of *Hepar sulphur* is to be preceded by a dose of *Pyrogenium 9C* two or three hours before.

Pyrogenium

This remedy is indicated for avoiding superinfection and can also be prescribed almost systematically. It is a nosode prepared from a septic autolysate of beef, pork, and human placenta, which causes a septic, febrile state when tested on animals.

Apart from the preceding case, prescribe in 9C, five pellets once a day, until the symptoms clear up.

Antimonium tartaricum

Weak or moist rale, betraying the presence of a large quantity of thick mucus in the bronchi and lungs which makes **expectoration difficult. The dyspnea is pronounced and noisy**, with the sides of the nose quivering. The skin is pale and cold with sometimes **cyanosis of the lips and around the eyes,** which is the sign of serious problems in the hematosis.

The patient is **dejected and sleepy**.

As for *Hepar sulphur*, the low dilutions favor expectoration and the high dilutions dry up the secretions.

Prescribe five pellets in 5C twice a day during the onset to facilitate expectoration, then prescribe in 15C to dry it up.

Blatta orientalis

This remedy is especially indicated in coughs caused by **dyspneic bronchitis** which resembles asthma, with gurgling and sibilant rale.

Prescribe five pellets in 5C every hour or every two hours depending on the seriousness of the symptoms. Increase interval with improvement.

Chamomilla

This remedy is indicated for **infantile bronchitis due to teething**. Febrile or not, the child is irritable, and calm when picked up. One cheek is red and hot, the other is pale and cold.

Prescribe in 9C, five pellets several times a day depending on the intensity of the respiratory signs and the frequency of the bouts of anger.

RESOLUTION PHASE

While the fever is entering the lysis phase, the cough improves but persists along with the expectoration. To hasten recovery the following should be considered at this stage:

Pulsatilla

Dry cough at night compelling the patient to sit up, and **phlegm-producing cough during the day**, with thick, yellowish mucus. Improvement with movement and fresh air.

Sulphur iodatum

Tiring, violent cough which produces profuse, thick mucus which is difficult to expel. The patient needs fresh air.

In practice, the last two remedies can be prescribed systematically when acute bronchitis is abating. Indeed, they seem to encourage an emollient, decongestant, and anti-inflammatory reaction which corresponds to the physiopathologic needs encountered at the end of acute infections in the respiratory mucous membranes.

Therefore, during the abatement of such diseases one could always prescribe for one week, for example:

- *Pulsatilla 9* or *15C*: five pellets on awakening and at about five in the afternoon (for children prone to otitis, prescribe in 15C preferably);
- *Sulphur iodatum 9* or *15C*: five pellets at bedtime.

•••••••••

ACUTE PNEUMONOPATHY

Acute pneumonopathy is an infection of the pulmonary parenchyma due to viruses, related microorganisms, or bacteria.

We shall not touch upon the question of pulmonary suppuration, such as abscesses in the lungs, in which homeopathy can only play an adjuvant role, nor acute infantile pneumonopathy in cases which involve blood problems requiring intensive care.

The most exact diagnosis possible must be made based on:

- **the clinical signs**: febrile syndrome, respiratory functional signs (cough, expectoration, stitch in the side, etc.);
- **radiology**, which makes it possible to detect acute lobar pneumonia and more diffuse, less typical sorts of pneumonopathy;
- **biology**: blood count, bacteriology, and possibly serology.

The reactive potential of the patient should be evaluated and a factor of gravity based on his constitution noted: elderly, diabetic, alcoholic, patient suffering from respiratory insufficiency, heavy smoker, etc.

This account makes it possible to choose the better therapeutic strategy:

- **antibiotics**: for serious forms or for forms with a specific bacteriological type (in this case homeopathy is used while waiting for the laboratory results or as an adjuvant);
- **homeopathy**: especially in the viral forms and in the absence of bacterial superinfection.

The clinical picture is composed of fever, general signs, respiratory functional signs with a cough.

PERIOD OF ONSET

We see practically the same clinical forms as in the descriptions of remedies for acute bronchitis: *Aconitum* and *Belladonna* to which may be added *Oscillococcinum®* (one dose to be taken as soon as possible and to be repeated six to twelve hours later) given the effectiveness of this medicine in treating viral infections.

FULLY-DECLARED PHASE

It is important to distinguish the forms with or without expectoration and specific localization.

FORMS WITHOUT EXPECTORATION

Bryonia

There is **dryness of the mucous membranes** and sometimes there is already **serous exudation** (pleura) which corresponds to the second stage of the inflammation, with fever, sweating which brings relief, a **painful stitch in the side** aggravated by movement or respiration; **improvement with pressure, immobility**, or lying on the side which is painful. The **cough** is **dry**, and is aggravated on entering a warm bedroom.

Prescribe *Bryonia 9C*, five pellets two to four times a day.

Phosphorus

This remedy is indicated when the focus of congestion is clear. There is a high temperature with a burning sensation in the palms of the hands, **unquenchable thirst** for cold water, **variable dyspnea, and a painful, dry cough**. Aggravation from lying on the left side. The expectoration may be streaked with blood.

Prescribe *Phosphorus 9C*, one dose morning and evening. For **viral pulmonary infiltrates** with more discreet symptoms, most frequently diagnosed only from an X-ray, prescribe in 9 or 15C, every day or every two days until the X-ray image is clear. The similarity in this case is anatomicopathological (*Phosphorus* is contra-indicated for progressive pulmonary tuberculosis).

Arsenicum album

This remedy is prescribed on the notion of bronchial and pulmonary inflammation with the patient showing **precise general signs** which are characteristic of the proving of *Arsenicum album*:

- **serious infectious state**, with weakness, agitation, sensitivity to the cold;
- **burning pains** improved with heat;
- **thirst** for small quantities of cold water, at frequent intervals;
- **nocturnal aggravation between one and three in the morning**.

The pneumonopathy may be complicated by **dyspnea or asthma**.

Depending on the extent of the similarity, 9 or 15C is prescribed, once or twice a day, depending on the intensity of the symptoms.

FORMS WITH EXPECTORATION

Ipeca

Spasmodic cough with suffocation, accompanied by nausea and vomiting; **dyspneic, emetic cough**.

Sizable accumulation of mucus in the bronchi, with disseminated, fine rale.

The tongue remains clear or lightly coated. **Hypersalivation. No thirst**.

Prescribe five pellets in 9C two to four times a day depending on the intensity of the symptoms.

Antimonium tartaricum

Fine or moist rale, betraying the presence in the bronchi and lungs of a large quantity of thick mucus making **expectoration difficult. The dyspnea is intense and noisy** and the sides of the nose quiver. The skin is pale and cold, with sometimes **cyanosis in the lips and rings under the eyes**.

The patient is **dejected and sleepy**.

As in the case of *Hepar sulphur*, low dilutions encourage expectoration and high dilutions dry up the secretions.

Prescribe five pellets in 5C twice a day during the onset to facilitate expectoration, then prescribe in 15C to dry it up.

Hepar sulphur

With this remedy, the cough is first of all dry, and then there is a tendency towards suppuration with **profuse purulent expectoration** and moist rale.

Dosage

The action of *Hepar sulphur* with regard to suppuration depends on the strength of the dilution used:

- **The low dilutions** (5C) **enhance suppuration** and play a centrifugal role (as for low dilutions of *Sulphur*, there is a possible aggravation of suppuration in an enclosed cavity: e.g. otitis). In 5C *Hepar sulphur* favors expectoration at the onset. Prescribe five pellets twice a day.
- **The high dilutions** (15-30C) **check suppuration**. *Hepar sulphur* 15C dries up the expectoration. Prescribe five pellets once to twice a day.

Pyrogenium

To prevent superinfection *Pyrogenium 9C* may be almost systematically prescribed in this case too, five pellets once a day.

THE FACTOR OF LOCALIZATION

Depending on the localization of the pulmonary complaints, some remedies are more specifically indicated according to the affinity revealed during the provings for such or such a pulmonary region.

Aviaire

Aviaire is the tuberculin of birds, obtained from antiseptic-free cultures of Mycobacterium tuberculosis of avian origin.

This remedy is indicated for complaints located **at the top of the lungs**, especially in children.

Prescribe a single dose in 15C, not to be repeated. Give the dose when the body temperature is at its highest. This remedy is also useful for recurrent pneumonopathy and otitis (*Homeopathic Therapeutics: Possibilities in chronic pathology)*.

• • • • • • • • •

Some authors recommend *Natrum sulphuricum* and *Antimonium sulphur aureum* for the forms of bronchopneumopathy occurring in the left base and *Kali carbonicum* for those in the right base of the lung.

We consider these to be more remedies to be recommended for chronic complaints.

COMMENT

If the reactive mode of the patient corresponds to two or three of the remedies described above, it is altogether **possible and proper** to prescribe them alternately in the same day.

RESOLUTION PHASE

As in the case of acute bronchitis and for the same physiopathologic reasons, the following may be prescribed systematically at this clinical stage for one week:

- *Pulsatilla 9* or *15C*, five pellets on awakening and about five in the afternoon (for children subject to otitis, prefer 15C);
- *Sulphur iodatum 9* or *15C*, five pellets at bedtime.

NON-PURULENT ACUTE PLEURISY

Pleurisy or pleuritis is an inflammation of the pleura with or without effusion.

When non-purulent acute pleurisy is diagnosed, it is a good idea to carry out the etiology:
- case history;
- blood count, ESR;
- intradermal reaction to tuberculin;
- biology: chemistry, cytology, bacteriology of the puncture fluid.

Indeed, homeopathic treatment will only be possible for **non-purulent infectious serofibrinous pleurisy and traumatic pleurisy**. All the other causes (tuberculosis, pulmonary embolism, cancer or cancerous metastasis, subdiaphragmatic complaints, etc.) will require the appropriate allopathic treatment, homeopathy in these cases serving only as an adjuvant.

The homeopathic treatment will consist of prescribing in hahnemannian dilutions the substances whose provings in the healthy person caused pleural irritation and a global reactive mode similar to those observed in the patient.

PERIOD OF ONSET

In the case of an infectious cause the remedies for the first stage in inflammation, described elsewhere, are available: *Aconitum, Belladonna, Ferrum phosphoricum,* since their prescription prevents the effusion from taking place.

During the fully-declared phase, the symptomatology becomes characteristic and corresponds to the following remedies:

FULLY-DECLARED PHASE

Bryonia

This is the principal remedy for this disease, corresponding to the most frequent cases. The fever is light, and continuous or remittent. The patient is dejected and tired; **he tries to remain immobile and is intensely thirsty**.

The painful stitch in the side is aggravated by movement and by breathing; **it is improved by applying pressure and remaining still** or lying on the side that is painful. There may also be a little **dry, painful cough, provoked by the slightest movement**.

The auscultation and the clinical examination reveal either pleural friction which means dry pleurisy or clear signs of effusion.

Prescribe *Bryonia* 15C, one dose every twelve hours.

Apis mellifica

The fever is not very high. There is dyspnea aggravated by heat; the cough is aggravated by lying down, and at night.

The thoracic pain is stinging, burning, **aggravated by heat**. The patient presents phases during which the skin is dry and hot, alternating with sweating phases.

Oliguria and absence of thirst.

Prescribe five pellets in 9 or 15C every six hours.

Cantharis

The provings have shown evidence of an action on the serous membranes. *Cantharis* is indicated when the effusion is profuse and accompanied by burning pains which are **improved by heat**. The dry cough has no characteristic modality.

There may be **oliguria**.

Prescribe *Cantharis 9C*, five pellets two to four times a day. When the pleural effusion is associated with obvious signs of oliguria, *Cantharis* may be alternated with *Apis* since both remedies have shown a common affinity during provings for the serous membranes and the renal parenchyma.

Arnica

This remedy corresponds as much to serofibrinous as to serous and hematic effusion following **direct or indirect traumatism** (post-commissurotomy syndrome, and Dressler's post-infarction syndrome which begin with pericardial effusion).

Depending on the symptoms, it may be used in 9 or 15C in conjunction with one of the preceding remedies.

RESOLUTION PHASE

The following is prescribed during the resolution phase for any type of serofibrinous pleurisy to facilitate convalescence:

Sulphur iodatum

Because of its affinity during provings for the serous membranes, this remedy enhances the resorption of the effusion and prevents adhesion from taking place.

Prescribe *Sulphur iodatum 9C*, five pellets per day, then one dose three times a week.

As a conclusion, it should be remembered that in the treatment of non-purulent acute pleurisy, the homeopathic treatment has only a modest place today. But it must be emphasized that its systematic prescription, as an adjuvant to conventional therapy, has nevertheless the advantage of reducing the progression time and preventing pleural adhesion from developing.

CHAPTER IV

DIGESTIVE TRACT

ACUTE STOMATOLOGY: PAIN - HEMORRHAGE - INFECTION

Homeopathy can be effective for several stomatological problems:

- preparation of a patient for dental surgery;
- prevention and treatment of post-operative hemorrhaging;
- prevention and treatment of infection, post-operative or not;
- toothache, especially when post-operative;
- as a complement to the treatment of wisdom teeth problems.

PRE-OPERATIVE CARE

Some patients are worried before undergoing dental surgery. Their reactive mode may indicate the prescription of *Gelsemium* or *Ignatia* (see "Pre and Post-Surgery Care" p. 117). Other patients may benefit from:

Chamomilla

This remedy is often indicated for teething infants; it is also indicated for **temperamental, irascible, highly strung adults who cannot tolerate pain**.

Odontalgia is **aggravated by heat, but not relieved by cold**.

Prescribe five pellets in 9, 15, or 30C generally once or twice a day, for a few days before and after surgery.

Coffea tosta

This remedy is indicated for intelligent, **nervous individuals**, who show signs of **mental overactivity** and are prone to insomnia (due to nervous anticipation). Fear of pain, and pain itself, makes them so agitated that they shake.

The odontalgia corresponding to *Coffea* is **relieved by contact with cold water**.

Same dosage as *Chamomilla*.

POST-OPERATIVE HEMORRHAGING

Arnica

This remedy is indicated since there is traumatism following the extraction of the capillaries. **Prescribing it systematically** limits hemorrhaging, accelerates resorption of edema, and therefore facilitates cicatrization and relieves pain.

Prescribe five daily pellets in 9C three days before surgery, then five pellets two to six times a day after surgery, depending on the intensity of the bleeding.

Phosphorus

This is a homeopathic remedy which prevents hemorrhaging; it is administered systematically the day before and on the morning of surgery, a dose in 9C every time.

If abnormal bleeding occurs despite these two remedies, the following remedies will be combined with *Arnica* and *Phosphorus*:

China

If the hemorrhage is of **black or dark blood**, prescribe five pellets in 5C every half-hour or every hour, alternating with *Arnica*. Increase interval with improvement.

Millefolium

Use if the hemorrhage is of fluid, **bright, red blood** and is hardly painful or not painful at all. It is also a good remedy for patients with a tendency to bleed profusely at the slightest cut (with no signs of hemopathy) or for women with profuse menstruation and the characteristics described above.

Same dosage as for *China*.

In these cases of abnormal hemorrhaging, the prescription of *Phosphorus* in 9 or 15C can also be repeated, a dose every six hours approximately.

POST-OPERATIVE OR NON POST-OPERATIVE INFECTIONS

Two remedies must be systematically prescribed to avoid risks of infection: *Pyrogenium* and *Hepar sulphur*.

They are complemented by *Arsenicum album, Aurum muriaticum, Mercurius solubilis,* or *Apis*, according to the patient's reactive modalities.

Pyrogenium

This nosode may be prescribed as a preventive measure before the operation if there is the risk of an underlying infectious focus: prescribe five pellets in 9C in the mornings and evenings of the two days preceding the operation.

As a curative measure, prescribe five pellets morning and evening in 9C followed by *Hepar sulphur* two hours later, for three or four days.

Hepar sulphur

This major homeopathic remedy for acute suppuration is prescribed in high dilutions, since conversely low dilutions encourage suppuration. Five pellets in 15 or 30C, for example, can be prescribed morning and evening for three or four days.

In addition, combine one of the following remedies with it:

Arsenicum album

In the case of burning, intense pain, relieved by applying anything warm. In addition, the discharge may be serous, bloody, purulent, but always extremely nauseating and excoriating.

The patient may be dejected and **tired because of the infectious process** which affects his overall condition profoundly; he is intensely thirsty. But these general symptoms are not essential for the prescription of the remedy.

According to similarity, prescribe in 9 or 15C, five pellets twice a day, at about 10 a.m. and 5 p.m.

Aurum muriaticum

For the reasons already mentioned on p. 96, this remedy is preferable to *Aurum metallicum* for suppuration in short bones in general, and suppurative processes of the jaw in particular.

Prescribe in at least 9C, five pellets at about 10 a.m. and 5 p.m.

Mercurius solubilis

This remedy is prescribed when the **characteristic buccopharyngeal signs** are present:

- whitish or yellowish, viscous, **thick tongue** which **shows marks of the teeth** (along the sides or if the tongue is bitten);
- **stringy**, nauseating **saliva**, and **intense thirst**;
- **spongy, bleeding gums**.

Prescribe in 9 or 15C, five pellets at about 10 a.m. and 5 p.m., since low dilutions may encourage suppuration.

Apis mellifica

This remedy is prescribed in the case of a marked **edematous reaction**, as is often the case in inflammatory processes in the mouth.

Prescribe five pellets in 15C every 30 to 60 minutes, increasing the interval with improvement.

When the constituted purulent collection can be easily drained, *Hepar sulphur 5C* and *Mercurius solubilis 5C* are prescribed to speed up maturation: five pellets alternately every four to six hours, for example, until incision or spontaneous bursting of the abscess.

The patient should also rinse his mouth out several times a day with thirty drops of a mixture of equal parts of *Phytolacca MT* - *Calendula MT* in half a glass of water.

TOOTHACHE

Several cases may be observed:
- toothache of surgical origin;
- infectious or inflammatory toothache;
- dental neuralgia, which is often paroxysmal, at the level of the trigeminal nerve in the lower or upper jawbone.

Etiologic treatment should be used when possible; but also think of:

Arnica

This remedy has an affinity for the capillaries; it is effective for pain after dental extraction, and also in dental neuralgia, in 9C, associated with:

Hypericum perforatum

This is the remedy for traumatism in nerve endings. The pain spreads along the path of the nerve concerned. It is nagging, unbearable, and worsened by even the slightest jolt.

Prescribe in 15 or 30C, depending on the frequency of the painful paroxysms.

Mezereum

This remedy experimentally causes an **irritation of the mucous membranes and of the periosteum**, principally at the level of the **malar regions**; therefore, it can also have an analgesic indication in stomatology.

It is specially effective **when the pain is due to superinfection**.

Prescribe in 5C, five pellets two to four times a day.

• • • • • • • • •

If the pain displays clear modalities or characteristics which point toward the proving of one of the following remedies, this remedy should be prescribed:

Aconitum

Pain after **sudden chill**, aggravated around midnight by intense and sudden cold.

Belladonna

Throbbing pain, with dryness of the mucous membranes at the onset of an inflammatory process.

Apis

Burning and stinging pain, relieved by cold, with inflammatory edema.

Arsenicum album

Burning pain, relieved by heat.

Coffea tosta or Pulsatilla

Pain relieved by contact with cold water.

Chamomilla

Pain aggravated by heat but not improved by cold.

Cheiranthus

This remedy is useful in 30C, a dose every six to twelve hours in the case of **trismus** due to a buccopharyngeal complaint, and in particular, due to problems with the wisdom teeth.

• • • • • • • • •

TEETHING

Teething may cause a certain number of local or general problems in infants or young children.

At the local level, the following signs can sometimes be observed:

- **pericoronitis** with inflammation of the mucous membrane, hypersalivation, and effects on mood (agitation, insomnia); there may even be suppuration;
- **gingivitis**;
- **follicular cyst** with tumefaction of the marginal gingiva.

At the general level, concomitantly, the following signs may be observed:

- salivary and/or nasal hypersecretion;
- redness of the cheeks, or, more frequently, of only one cheek; eczema of the cheeks or diaper rash;
- rise in temperature;
- reflex otalgia;
- digestive phenomena: anorexia, vomiting, diarrhea, etc.;
- emotional behavior disorders: agitation, anger, insomnia.

A certain number of medicinal substances cause similar symptoms during their proving. Therefore, they are the corresponding homeopathic remedies.

AT THE LOCAL LEVEL

Borax

This is for gingivitis or stomatitis **with aphtae**; these lesions are very painful at the slightest contact, especially of acid or salty food. The baby cannot suck and refuses the breast or the bottle.

Prescribe *Borax 5C*, five pellets three or four times a day. This remedy is also suitable for candidiasis of the oral mucosa in infants (thrush).

In this particular case, it is recommended to also rinse the mouth with bicarbonated water so as to alkalinize the oral environment, and to prescribe a daily dose of *Candida albicans 15C* or a nosode for mycotic aphtae (*Homeopathic Therapeutics: Possibilities in chronic pathology*, chapter V).

Phytolacca

The infant has a compulsive urge to rub his gums together when teething.

Prescribe in 7C, five pellets, three or four times a day.

Mercurius solubilis

This remedy is indicated when there is inflammation of the gums accompanied by **hypersalivation and a thick, swollen tongue**. There is sometimes concomitant **stomatitis**. The young patient is **intensely thirsty**.

Prescribe in 9C, five pellets once or twice a day.

AT THE GENERAL LEVEL

In the presence of general or concomitant symptoms, the principal remedy for teething should be considered:

Chamomilla

The proving reveals **hyperesthesia to pain, an irritable, irascible, capricious mood, digestive disorders**.

Chamomilla is indicated for the capricious, irascible baby who is tired out by his teething.

Very often **one cheek is red and warm, the other pale and cold**.

The child's bad moods are **improved when he is picked up and carried** or taken for a drive.

During teething, there may also be: hyperthermia, diarrhea, or bronchitis.

Dosage

For the infant who is usually pleasant and well-behaved but becomes irascible with painful teething, give five pellets of *Chamomilla 15C*, to be repeated every quarter of an hour if necessary. Relief is generally rapid. Stop the remedy as soon as the pain is relieved.

Apart from mood disorders, when there is also fever, diarrhea, or coughing, prescribe *Chamomilla 15C*, five pellets twice a day, possibly in association with the necessary complementary homeopathic remedy, depending on symptomatology. In particular:

Podophyllum

In the case of copious **aqueous and mucous diarrhea**, preceded by pain and borborygmi.

Diarrhea is **more frequent in the morning**, and the pain is **improved when the child is lying on his stomach**.

The infant squeezes his gums.

Prescribe *Podophyllum* in 9 or 15C, five pellets after each bowel movement: lower dilutions may maintain or aggravate the diarrheic phenomena.

Medorrhinum

This remedy is indicated in the case of diaper rash for an infant who tends to sleep with his knees folded up to his chest.

Prescribe in 9 or 15C, one or two doses a week.

HEPATIC COLIC

Hepatic colic is characterized by sharp pain at the level of the right hypochondrium, spreading to the epigastrium and to the back, often associated with nausea and vomiting. It is linked with an acute distention of the bile ducts.

The principal cause of hepatic colic is biliary lithiasis, which is responsible for about 98% of the cases. But other possible causes must not be ignored: cancer (especially Vater's ampulla carcinoma), benign tumors, choledochitis, certain types of parasitosis (fluke, ascariasis, and especially a hydatid cyst which breaks in the bile ducts).

Here hepatic colic of lithiasic origin is being dealt with.

In hyperalgesic hepatic colic attacks, conventional antispasmodic medicines are obviously capable of relieving the patient very rapidly. Homeopathic treatment is then only a complement, but it may be enough on its own for certain mild or medium crises.

Belladonna

Pain starts and ends abruptly; it is aggravated by the slightest touch, even by stroking, and by jolting. The abdomen is tense and warm. General signs are often present: fever and cephalic congestion. If an emergency surgical operation is ruled out, prescribe *Belladonna* in 9 or 15C, five pellets depending on the frequency of the painful crises.

It is often beneficial to alternate this remedy with one of the following medicines, which are indicated by the patient's reactive symptoms.

Colocynthis

Pain is spasmodic and violent; it starts and ends abruptly. The patient feels better doubled up, with heat and pressure: **lying curled up is particularly good for relieving the pain**.

Prescribe five pellets in 9 or 15C every ten to fifteen minutes, increasing the interval with improvement.

Dioscorea villosa

This remedy is indicated in the same dosage as *Colocynthis* for patients whose modality for relieving the paroxysmal pain is the opposite of *Colocynthis*: **relief by arching the back**. It is much less often indicated.

Bryonia alba

This is the remedy for inflammation of the serous membranes and of the parenchyma of the organs they surround. *Bryonia* is prescribed according to the following reactive modalities:

- **stinging, nagging pain** in the hepatobiliary region, **caused or aggravated by even slight**

movement, by breathing in deeply; the patient is relieved by lying on his right side and by widely-applied pressure;
- continuous or remittent **fever**, accompanied by **intense thirst for large quantities of cold water** at long intervals, oily perspiration which brings relief;
- bitter taste in the mouth, white tongue, dry lips;
- hard, dry, black, voluminous stools, more frequently encountered than bilious diarrhea with the slightest movement.

Prescribe in 5 to 15C, according to similarity, five pellets every two hours. Increase interval with improvement.

Berberis vulgaris

There is very acute, paroxysmal pain, like the stab of a dagger; it radiates from a precise point to the stomach and the abdomen; it is aggravated by slow or sudden movement, like the pain of *Bryonia;* it is also **aggravated by pressure**, unlike the pain of *Bryonia.*

A concomitant painful sensitivity to pressure is often observed at the level of the left lumbocostal angle; it can also be noticed that the urine varies considerably in quantity and concentration.

Prescribe five pellets in 5 to 9C three or four times a day.

Chamomilla

This remedy may be indicated for agitated and irascible **patients who have little tolerance for pain**.

Prescribe in 15 or 30C, five pellets three times a day.

Nux vomica

This remedy is prescribed according to the digestive signs observed (spasmodic pain, nausea, vomiting, pyrosis); but it is especially prescribed in relation to a particular constitution:
- hypersensitive, sedentary subject,
- usually inclined to good food and overeating.

Prescribe in 9 or 15C two to four times a day.

Ricinus communis

The hepatic colic is manifested by pain around the waist, accompanied by diarrhea.

Prescribe in 5C, alternately with *Belladonna*, depending on the frequency of the painful paroxysms.

Calcarea carbonica

This remedy is very effective in 15 or 30C for renal colic, but much less so in acute attacks of hepatic colic. However, it is a major constitutional remedy for biliary lithiasis *Homeopathic Therapeutics: Possibilities in chronic pathology*.

Therefore, homeopathic treatment can relieve a patient suffering from hepatic colic in a significant number of cases, associated or not with traditional antispasmodic medicines. Moreover, this method can be a treatment for lithiasic constitutions.
As for the few cases of hepatic colic which are not due to lithiasis, they require an etiologic treatment, most of the time surgical.

ACUTE HEPATITIS

Acute hepatitis corresponds to **histologic alterations of hepatocytes** whose complex physiopathology can be studied according to biological, immunologic, and etiologic clinical parameters.

Jaundice of cytolytic or cholestatic origin due to failure of the biliary function can usually be observed; it is not, however, a necessary characteristic of the complaint.

The cause of acute hepatitis must be determined in order to choose an adequate treatment, whether medicinal or surgical.

ETIOLOGY OF ACUTE HEPATITIS

Acute obstructions of the bile ducts within or outside the liver are not studied here: they require surgical treatment.

1. VIRAL HEPATITIS

These are the most common types. A number of viruses responsible has been distinguished:

- **type A, B, C, delta viruses**;
- **other viruses**: Epstein-Barr virus, cytomegalovirus, yellow fever flavivirus, coxsackievirus, herpesvirus, etc.

2. TOXIC HEPATITIS

This form of hepatitis is caused by several hepatotoxic pharmacodynamic substances which can lead to cytolysis or steatosis lesions or more rarely to cholangitis and pericholangitis, depending on the case:

- Amanita phalloides;
- solvents: nitric derivatives, halogen hydrocarbons;
- metals: mercury, lead, etc.
- medicines: paracetamol, chlorpromazine, antibiotics, MAO inhibitors, etc.

3. MICROBIAL HEPATITIS

This form is essentially an icteric manifestation which occurs either during septicemia, or during microbial infectious diseases: leptospirosis, brucellosis, typhoid and paratyphoid fever, etc.

The etiologic study enables the link to be established between hepatitis and homeopathic therapy. As Professor R. Brette[8] pointed out:

"There are many types of etiology of jaundice from hepatitis, with variable constitutional modes and clinical aspects. It sometimes looks cytolytic, sometimes has a cholestatic retention aspect. Viruses indifferently induce either form, but are more often cytolytic, just like toxic hepatitis, whereas many common medicines are the cause of cholestatic hepatitis.

In most cases, **an immune allergic mechanism seems to play a role in the appearance of lesions of the hepatocytes or the bile canaliculi, which explains the similarity of the clinical anatomical aspects produced by apparently very different etiologic agents".**

Since the anatomicopathological lesions observed in acute hepatitis are identical and the clinical signs are similar, whatever the cause of the hepatitis, homeopathic remedies are the same. All the conditions necessary for the choice of homeopathic treatment are indeed present :

1.- **the syndrome can be reversed** because the hepatocytes can regenerate;

2.- **there are pharmacodynamic substances which are able to induce**, in material doses, **similar anatomicopathological lesions**, whether they are cytolytic or cholestatic lesions.

In the range of homeopathic medicines available, some must be used **from the phase of onset** (in Caroli's triad when encountered): three principal remedies correspond to the **acute cytolytic phase**, whereas others are intended to correct the cholestasis and the hepatobiliary insufficiency which are the causes of the **accompanying digestive disorders**.

PERIOD OF ONSET OF VIRAL HEPATITIS (CAROLI'S TRIAD)

It is often preceded by a period of dysphagia; it combines **migrainous headache, urticaria, and arthralgia**.

Two medicines must be prescribed when it is observed:

Apis mellifica

The symptoms of the proving include:

- pruritic, burning, pinkish-red **edematous eruptions**, relieved by applying something cold;
- **articular pain**;
- **congestive headache**;
- **edema in the throat**.

(8) Brette R. et al., *Cahiers médicaux*, volume 3, n°30, 10 avril 1978; p.1792.

Bryonia alba

The symptoms of the proving include:

- migrainous **headache**, with nausea, a bitter taste in the mouth, constipation;
- **acute arthritis**.

It is also a remedy for an adynamic febrile syndrome with dryness of the mucous membranes.

Prescribe these two medicines in 9C, five pellets of each alternately, with an increased frequency if the symptoms are more marked.

REMEDIES OF THE FULLY-DECLARED PHASE (CYTOLYSIS REMEDIES)

Phosphorus

This is the key remedy for viral hepatitis. Apart from the fact that white phosphorus is one of the most powerful hepatotoxic substances and can therefore already be indicated because of the anatomicopathological similarity, the symptoms of the proving of *Phosphorus* include:

- a phase of agitation followed by **asthenia** and **vertigo**;
- **headache** with congestive flush;
- **hyperthermia** with a sensation of burning internal heat and profuse hot sweating;
- **digestive disorders** with a red and glossy tongue, intense thirst for cold water (often rejected soon after ingestion), nausea, gastralgia, painless copious diarrhea which burns the anus, or constipation;
- a congested, painful **enlarged liver** which is sensitive to touch and pressure;
- possible **jaundice**;
- tendency towards **hemorrhaging.**

Prescribe a unit-dose tube of *Phosphorus 9* or *15C* morning and evening for ten days, then in the morning only for another ten days. The following doses depend on an improvement in the results of the biological tests in general, and in the transaminase level in particular.

Arsenicum album

The proving of this substance also covers the symptoms of hepatitis:

- alternating phases of **agitation and prostration**;
- congestive and migrainous **headache** relieved by cold;
- **hyperthermia** with a sensation of burning and a desire for warmth;
- **digestive disorders** with vomiting and burning diarrhea, pain relieved by heat, intense thirst for small quantities of cold water;
- **a painful liver**;
- possible **jaundice**;
- tendency towards **anemia**;
- burning pruritus relieved by heat;
- aggravation of symptoms at night around 1 a.m.

But to complement this clinical picture, there is above all a **marked weakening asthenia** which causes **anxiety** in the patient.

Same dosage as for *Phosphorus*.

Mercurius solubilis

Weakness, asthenia, and anxiety dominate the clinical picture for *Arsenicum album*, whereas here digestive signs are the most obvious:

- **syndrome of gastroenteritis** with stomatitis: moist tongue which shows marks of the teeth, gingivitis, dysphagia, metallic taste, fetid breath, thirst, nausea, and blood-streaked, glairy diarrhea which causes irritation;
- **hyperthermia** with sweating which brings no relief;
- **painful right hypochondrium**, aggravated when lying on the right side;
- possible **jaundice**;
- **pruritus** aggravated in the warmth of the bed;
- **insomnia**.

Same dosage as *Phosphorus*.

COMPLEMENTARY REMEDIES

These are remedies for **cholestasis** and **hepatocellular insufficiency**. Their prescription is based on biological data (drop in the albumin level, decreased prothrombin time, increased bilirubinemia). The choice depends on the patient's clinical reactive symptoms.

We want to emphasize the fact that the following remedies are to be prescribed **in addition to** the previous ones, since they do not include phenomena of hepatic cytolysis in their proving:

Chelidonium majus

This is a good remedy for cholestasis, which is prescribed on the clinical notion of growing pain in the hepatic region **spreading to the tip of the right scapula**. A desire for warm food and drink, a saburral tongue, a bitter taste in the mouth, and fetid breath can also be noticed.

Prescribe in 4 or 5C, five pellets twice a day.

Lycopodium

This is the remedy of the hepatic cells and bile ducts and this affinity dominates its proving; it is prescribed for the following symptoms:

- sensitivity of the right hypochondrium (the patient **cannot lie on his right side**);
- **appetite quickly sated**;
- **postprandial bloating** especially under the umbilicus, with a peak around 4 or 5 p.m.;
- constipation with ineffective urges.

Prescribe in 5C, five pellets twice a day.

China rubra

This remedy is for hypertrophy of the liver and the spleen; it prevents hemorrhaging, corrects anemia, asthenia, and abdominal bloating with parietal hyperesthesia.

Prescribe five pellets in 5 or 7C twice a day.

Hydrastis canadensis

This remedy is indicated for jaundice which regresses slowly, intense constipation, and a weakened overall condition due to "a mucous plug in the bile ducts".

Prescribe five pellets in 4 or 5C twice a day.

•••••••••

Applied in this way, the homeopathic treatment for a patient with acute hepatitis causes a very fast regression of the clinical signs and normalization of the biological parameters in two or three weeks; it prevents subsequent asthenia and possible relapse.

•••••••••

CYCLIC VOMITING IN CHILDREN

This complaint is also called periodic ketosis, since vomiting is contingent.

Hyperketonemia is the consequence of a **transitory disturbance of the lipid metabolism** when there is a momentary shortage of available glucose following insufficient provision or excessive expenditure of carbohydrates:

- variations in diet (excess fats, simple fasting, carbohydrate fasting, diabetes),
- febrile reaction to an infectious or inflammatory process,
- intestinal parasitosis,
- physical overexertion,
- a tiring journey, change in climate or altitude,
- asthma, neurologic or endocrine diseases,
- emotion or upset.

Hepatic ketogenesis, which is the normal destination of acetyl CoA, reaches too high a level; acetoacetic acid, beta-hydroxybutyric acid, and ketone bodies accumulate in the blood, and ketonemia may reach a level of several grams per liter (physiologic rate: 15 to 20 mg/liter). They are then eliminated in the urine although ketonuria does not necessarily follow ketonemia.

The homeopathic treatment studied here is only for the simple attack of cyclic vomiting. We will not deal with diseases in which excess ketogenesis is only part of the problem (diabetes, hyperthyroidism, etc.)

On a clinical level, **vomiting**, of varying amounts but often containing bile, is accompanied by **abdominal pain**, **moderate metabolic fever**, **dejection**, a certain degree of **pallor** with rings around the eyelids, and an **aromatic odor on the breath** like the odor of apples. The diagnosis of hyperketonemia is confirmed by the **presence of ketone bodies in the urine** ascertained by an indicator.

Cyclic vomiting essentially occurs in the form of attacks, principally in non-pubescent children, **with a particular constitution**: easily-tired, emotional, thin children, with a capricious appetite, attracted by salty or spicy food, pork meat, and cheese, averse to sweet things except chocolate, often suffering from worms, with migrainous or dyspeptic parents. This disease is rarely observed in North America because of the eating habits there.

The homeopathic treatment of the attack should be complemented by a dietary prescription.

PRINCIPAL HOMEOPATHIC MEDICINES

Senna

Senna is the principal medicine because experimentally it causes digestive disorders which are exactly similar to those observed during the ketonemia attack:

- **aromatic odor of the breath**;
- **nausea, vomiting, colic, and flatulence**;
- **rapid exhaustion with pallor of the face**.

It should be almost systematically prescribed, five pellets in 5C repeated every half-hour or every hour depending on the severity of the case.

The doses can be alternated with one or more of the following remedies depending on the patient's reactive modalities.

Lycopodium clavatum

This is generally used as a constitutional remedy for this type of complaint; it is used here as a remedy for an acute attack in thin patients with a yellowish complexion, generally suffering from borborygmi with often painful intestinal flatulence, aggravated by starchy food, eggs, and chocolate.

The patients for whom this remedy is appropriate are also often nervous, with a tendency towards eczema, and often suffered from diaper rash before they were potty-trained.

Prescribe in 5, or 9C, five pellets two or three times a day.

Phosphorus

The vomiting is **copious and burning** for the mouth and the esophagus; it often contains bile. There is **moderate fever**, sweating, prostration. There is intense **thirst for cold water** but the drinks are quickly brought up again; the tongue is dry and red.

Prescribe in 9C, five pellets alternating with *Senna*.

Ipeca

This medicine is used for copious vomiting with a **clear or lightly coated tongue**, sialorrhea, and **lack of thirst**.

Prescribe five pellets in 9C, depending on the frequency of the vomiting.

Antimonium crudum

This remedy is prescribed in the case of copious food vomiting, accompanied by a **tongue covered with a chalk-white coating** and **intense thirst** mainly for acidic or effervescent drinks.

This clinical picture is generally observed in cyclic vomiting following overeating.

Same dosage as for *Ipeca*.

DIETARY PRESCRIPTION

There is glucose deficiency, as well as a loss of water and electrolytes. The patient must, therefore, be **abundantly** provided with:

- **water**,
- **carbohydrates**,
- **electrolytes** (mainly sodium chloride to combat hypochloremia).

To that effect abundant sweet drinks are recommended (herbal tea, fresh fruit juice, lemonade, soda) and salty vegetable broth. They must be ingested cold, lukewarm, or hot, in small frequently repeated quantities, depending on the patient's appetite and on how well he tolerates them.

Lipids and proteins, including dairy products, **must be absolutely eliminated** from the diet, until the ketonuria, monitored with an indicator, disappears.

Solid food then consists of bread, pasta, potatoes, carrots, flour-based food prepared with water, stewed fruit, and jam.

ACUTE GASTROENTERITIS IN INFANTS AND ADULTS

The clinical characteristic of acute gastroenteritis is the **combination of vomiting and diarrhea**. Vomiting is the sudden rejection of the gastric contents by antiperistaltic contractions; diarrhea is over-frequent evacuation of stools which are too liquid.

Diarrhea is due to a double mechanism generally occurring at the same time:

- **acceleration of the intestinal passage**,
- **abnormal hydration of stools by hypersecretion of the intestinal mucous membrane**.

These mechanisms are the direct consequences of an attack on the digestive mucosa.

Acute gastroenteritis is not a nosologically-defined autonomous disease; it is only a reactive syndrome which can be observed in an often complex clinical set of symptoms, resulting from various causes:

- various food toxic infections;
- seasonal digestive problems;
- infectious diseases (typhoid, cholera, influenza, otitis, etc.).

Diarrhea and vomiting may or may not be associated; when profuse, they cause metabolic disorders. Given the digestive affinity of many pharmacodynamic substances, homeopathic medicines are particularly numerous.

For didactic reasons, five different cases have been distinguished:

- isolated acute gastroenteritis,
- febrile acute gastroenteritis,
- acute gastroenteritis with dehydration,
- acute gastroenteritis in infants,
- remedies for convalescence after acute gastroenteritis.

In each case, only the most reliable and most often encountered medicines are studied. Medium or high dilutions should always be prescribed in order to dry up the secretions.

ISOLATED ACUTE GASTROENTERITIS

The patient displays either diarrhea, or vomiting, or a combination of diarrhea and vomiting with possible abdominal pain of variable intensity.

1. DIARRHEA DOMINANT

The choice of medicine can be rapidly pinpointed through the characteristic modalities of the diarrhea.

1. PROFUSE DIARRHEA

Podophyllum peltatum

The diarrhea is watery or mucous, **very copious**, preceded by pain and borborygmi. It occurs mainly **early in the morning** or before midday.
Stools are fetid, yellowish, ejected in a spurt, **followed by tenesmus**, **extreme weakness**, and a sensation of emptiness in the abdomen.
Pain is **relieved** by heat and **by lying on the stomach**.
Prescribe five pellets of *Podophyllum* after each bowel movement, at least in 9C, since low dilutions may aggravate the diarrhea.

Aloe socotrina

The diarrhea is copious, often mucous **like jelly**, accompanied by **a lot of intestinal wind** which the patient does not dare emit because the **sphincters are highly unreliable**. There may be a bowel movement immediately after a drink.
Prescribe in 9C, five pellets after each bowel movement.

2. PAINFUL DIARRHEA

Magnesia phosphorica

This remedy is indicated when the diarrhea is accompanied by **acute, cramp-like pain, with a sudden onset and end. Improvement** can be observed when the patient is **doubled up, and with heat and strong pressure**.

Prescribe in 9C, in time with the pain and/or bowel movements.

Colocynthis

Since magnesium phosphate is one of the pharmacodynamic constituents of colocynth, *Magnesia phosphorica* and *Colocynthis* can be used indifferently.

Cuprum metallicum and Cuprum sulphuricum

During tests, copper causes gastroenteritis with spasmodic signs occurring in both smooth and striated muscles; copper sulfate has proved to be a powerful laxative.

In homeopathic therapeutics, these remedies are indicated for violent diarrhea accompanied by **cramp-like pain** in the whole abdomen and even in the calves. Pain **starts and ends abruptly**. The patient may also feel intermittent stomach cramps which may be very violent, with nausea and vomiting; all these signs are temporarily **relieved** by **drinking one or more mouthfuls of cold water**.

Prescribe five pellets in 9C depending on the frequency of the bowel movements and/or painful cramps.

Cambogia or Gambogia

The diarrhea is **preceded by noisy borborygmi** and **periumbilical pain**; it appears as **sudden, pressing, painful urge**, followed by a yellowish stool **emitted in a single, prolonged jet** which brings **general relief**. It is aggravated by absorbing food and drinks.

Its indication, in general, tends to be encountered more in adults, and in elderly people in particular.

Same dosage as *Cuprum*.

3. PAINLESS DIARRHEA

China rubra

This remedy is indicated in the presence of:
- **distention of the whole abdomen** (which the patient seems to contain with his hands), **with marked flatulence**;
- **tympanites** with percussion;
- **hypersensitivity to touching or stroking**.

Expulsion of stools is **painless**, but accompanied by a **sensation of fainting**. Everything tastes bitter.

The remedy is indicated after excesses of fruit or milk (and also in diarrhea in infants due to intolerance of gluten).

Prescribe *China 9C* after every bowel movement.

Ricinus communis

The diarrhea is watery, whitish, and resembles rice. Expulsion of stools is **painless**, preceded by **painless borborygmi**, accompanied by **numerous bouts of nausea**.

Same dosage as for *China*.

4. ANALLY EXCORIATING DIARRHEA

Croton tiglium

The diarrhea indicating *Croton* has four specific characteristics:
- it is **excoriating for the anus** and the perianal region;
- it is **liquid and yellow**;
- it is **expelled in a jet** with a noisy bang, like a gun shot;
- it is **caused by the ingestion of the slightest amount of food or drink**.

These modalities are often encountered in diarrhea resulting from treatment with antibiotics.

Prescribe five pellets in 9C depending on the frequency of the bowel movements.

Arsenicum album

A burning abdominal pain, relieved by local heat accompanies **liquid and blackish diarrhea which burns the anus and has a nauseating odor**.

Same dosage.

5. MOTOR DIARRHEA

In this case *Gelsemium sempervirens* or *Argentum nitricum* are indicated; these medicines are studied in the chapter "Nervous Apprehensiveness - Acute Reactive Emotional Disorders" p. 109.

2. VOMITING DOMINANT

In most cases, indigestion is due to overeating or to acute alcoholism.

Nux vomica

This medicine contains strychnine and brucine which are experimentally responsible for antiperistaltic spasms; it is used for **nausea, regurgitation, and acidic vomiting** which brings relief, following excessive eating or drinking.

Prescribe five pellets of *Nux vomica 9C* in time with the bouts of nausea. Using this medicine as a preventive measure, five pellets or a unit-dose tube before indulging in drinking episodes, facilitates digestion, diminishes the sensation of intoxication, and avoids the unpleasant sensation of "hangover" the following morning.

Antimonium crudum

This medicine is used for **eructation** with the **taste of food** for individuals who complain of sensations of **gastric fullness and heaviness**, due to the **gluttonous absorption** of a large amount of food.

The tongue is often markedly coated, covered with a **milk-white, thick coating**.

Soon afterwards **nausea** occurs, followed by **vomiting containing pieces of food**. The stools have a semi-solid, semi-liquid aspect.

Same dosage as for *Nux vomica*.

Ipeca

Here, the patient presents **vomiting** which does not relieve **his continual nausea. The tongue is clear or lightly coated**, and kept moist all the time by **hypersalivation**. The patient **does not feel thirsty**.

The stools are accompanied by **tenesmus**. They may be **fermented, green**, frothy, and **sometimes bloody**.

Prescribe five pellets of *Ipeca 9C*, repeated with increasing frequency according to the degree of severity of the symptoms.

FEBRILE ACUTE GASTROENTERITIS

Febrile acute gastroenteritis includes toxic food infections and "intestinal flu".

Aconitum napellus

After a **sudden chill, green diarrhea** occurs in an infant, a child, or an adult, sometimes accompanied by blood-stained mucus. **Hyperthermia** also occurs suddenly; the patient **does not sweat,** he is **agitated**, anxious, and **intensely thirsty** for cold water.

Prescribe five pellets in 9C after every bowel movement.

Arsenicum album

Burning abdominal pains, alleviated by the local application of heat, appear along with **blackish and liquid diarrhea which burns the anus; this diarrhea has a nauseating odor and exhausts the patient**. There is also **burning vomiting** and an **intense thirst** for cold water which is regurgitated soon after.

This clinical picture evolves in an **acute febrile context**, with sensitivity to cold, and **alternating phases of agitation and prostration**.

The disorders **are aggravated at night** between one and three in the morning.

These signs are generally observed in toxic infectious syndromes and *Arsenicum album* is an excellent remedy for **intoxication with food that has gone bad**: spoilt fish or meat, contaminated shellfish, polluted water.

Prescribe in 9C, five pellets repeated every hour, progressively increasing the interval between doses as symptoms diminish. This is a fast-acting medicine.

Dulcamara

The diarrhea is preceded by **borborygmi** and **periumbilical pain,** relieved by emitting wind; it **resembles diarrhea caused by dysentery**, and is either watery with sometimes blood-stained mucus, or mucous, viscous, green, or yellowish. It generally occurs in a **subacute febrile context** with **shivering**, following a **chill in damp weather**.

Same dosage as for *Arsenicum album*.

Mercurius solubilis

This remedy is indicated when the **stools** are **greenish, blood-stained**, or viscous, **worse at night, with tenesmus** and the impression that the expulsion will never end.

But the main sign is that the intestinal condition is **concomitant with buccopharyngeal** and overall **signs** which are characteristic of *Mercurius solubilis*:

- **fetid breath** with a metallic odor which spreads throughout the room;
- swollen, **flaccid tongue**, which retains the mark of the teeth along the sides, covered with a yellowish white viscous coating caused by excessive salivation which runs onto the pillow at night without relieving the intense thirst also experienced;
- **the fever is high**, stable, accompanied by shivering on the surface of the skin and sweating mainly at night which does not afford any relief.

Same dosage.

Mercurius corrosivus

This remedy is very similar to *Mercurius solubilis*. It is preferred to the latter for **subacute dysentery with even more painful tenesmus** than in the previous description.

The stools are **small, burning, blood-streaked or bloody,** with mucous lumps and **violent intestinal tormina**.

Same dosage.

ACUTE GASTROENTERITIS WITH DEHYDRATION

Severe choleriform diarrhea is responsible for dehydration with deterioration of the overall condition. Three successive stages can be observed:

- first of all, there is an expulsion of profuse stools which causes a loss of water and electrolytes;
- next, when the stools become scarcer, the patient becomes weaker and the pain increases;

- finally, when the patient can no longer eliminate anything, he feels a cramp-like pain.

These three phases correspond to three specific homeopathic medicines which can be used separately or in succession and thus make it possible to reverse a disquieting situation(9) (10). If necessary, rehydration and a correction of the electrolytic disorder must be ensured parenterally.

Veratrum album

This remedy is indicated in the case of **profuse**, febrile, **extremely copious diarrhea**, with cramp-like pain, **extreme prostration and abundant cold sweating**, principally on the forehead.

Associated vomiting is often copious and aggravates the tendency to collapse. The patient has a sensation of intense burning with **general cold throughout the body** and cyanosis in the extremities.

Prescribe five pellets of *Veratrum album 9C*, repeated very hour or depending on the frequency of the bowel movements, then increase the interval as symptoms become less intense.

Arsenicum album

This remedy is indicated when the **stools,** which **burn** like fire, **excoriate** the anus, and are **nauseating**, become **scarce**. They are often associated with the **burning vomiting** of the small amount of food the patient absorbs.

The patient is **febrile, extremely thirsty, very weak,** and displays **anxious agitation and dejection in turn**. The symptomatology involves nocturnal recrudescence, between 1 and 3 a.m.

Same dosage as for *Veratrum album*.

Cuprum metallicum

The patient now displays **cramp-like pain** over the whole of the abdomen and even in the calves, **with a sudden onset and end**, which are temporarily alleviated by absorbing a little cold water.

Same dosage.

ACUTE GASTROENTERITIS IN INFANTS

A certain number of medicines are more particularly used for infants. They are prescribed under specific conditions: teething, intolerance to milk, febrile acute gastroenteritis. Homeopathic remedies for toxicosis are indistinguishable from those studied in the section on acute gastroenteritis with dehydration.

(9) Thesis by Dr. Anne Guilly, Pascal Jandeaux, *Homéopathie et choléra au XIXe siècle*, Lille, 1985.

(10) Lucile Lasveaux, *Traitements homéopathiques du choléra dans la France du XIXème* - Boiron, France, 1985, 20 p.

1. ACUTE GASTROENTERITIS CONCOMITANT WITH TEETHING

Chamomilla vulgaris

Diarrhea and teething can be observed; the infant is **capricious, irascible, odious**, he can only be pacified by being picked up and carried continually or taken out in a car. The diarrhea is green, like spinach mixed with scrambled eggs. In the case of fever, one cheek is red and warm, whereas the other is pale and cold.

Because the infant's usual behavior is altered, prescribe five pellets of *Chamomilla 9* or *15C*, in timing with the painful bowel movements or the fits of anger.

Rheum officinale

The rhizome of rhubarb induces intestinal hypersecretion in experimental conditions. In homeopathic therapeutics, it is used for **teething infants** who are capricious and agitated, with profuse sweating on the scalp which gives off a **sour odor** despite all the efforts to keep the children clean.

Another therapeutic indication is diarrhea following excessive ingestion of unripe fruit.

Prescribe five pellets of *Rheum officinale 9C* depending on the frequency of the bowel movements.

Mercurius solubilis

With infants, this remedy is used during teething when a febrile syndrome, diarrhea, and **sialorrhea** are observed.

Prescribe in 9C, five pellets two to four times every twenty-four hours.

2. ACUTE GASTROENTERITIS DUE TO INTOLERANCE OF MILK

Magnesia carbonica

This remedy is for infants whose whole body gives off a sour odor and who cannot tolerate milk well. The diarrhea is watery, green, frothy, **like frog spawn**, with a sourish odor.

Prescribe in 9C depending on the frequency of the bowel movements.

3. FEBRILE GASTROENTERITIS

Apparently isolated, febrile acute gastroenteritis in infants is often concomitant with otitis. Homeopathic treatment consists then of the range of pharmacodynamic substances whose proving targets are the digestive and the ENT apparatus: *Aconitum, Chamomilla, Arsenicum album, Belladonna, Capsicum, Dulcamara, Mercurius solubilis* (see chapter on "Acute Otitis" p. 131).

CONVALESCENCE REMEDIES IN ACUTE GASTROENTERITIS

Acute gastroenteritis is an episode which often leaves two types of more or less temporary sequelae, once the acute attacks of digestive disorders are over:
- physical asthenia, and
- persistent soft or diarrheic stools with the slightest change in diet.

1. PERSISTENT ASTHENIA

China rubra

This remedy corresponds to **physical asthenia** with pallor and hypotension which can be found in patients who have suffered from abundant loss of organic fluids.

Prescribe five pellets of *China 9C* twice a day until the symptoms disappear, which is generally about ten days.

Natrum muriaticum

For infants or young children who often display severe asthenia and a marked loss of weight after episodes of diarrhea, *China rubra* is well complemented by one or two weekly doses of *Natrum muriaticum 9* or *15C* until the patient returns to his initial weight.

2. PERSISTENT SOFT STOOLS

Paratyphoidinum B and Eberthinum

These nosodes are prepared from antiseptic-free lysates obtained from the corresponding Salmonella cultures.

These two medicines may be indicated either on the basis of an etiologic indication, or on the clinical indication of persistent soft stools with the slightest change in diet following acute gastroenteritis. Pathologically, and therefore experimentally, these germs are actually responsible for irritation of the intestinal tract with diarrhea.

Prescribe a weekly dose in 9 or 15C until the symptoms improve.

CHAPTER V

URINARY TRACT PREGNANCY

ACUTE CYSTITIS

Cystitis is an **inflammation of the bladder** identifiable clinically as a syndrome consisting of:

- **pollakiuria**,
- **dysuria** (before, during, or after urination),
- **irrepressible and scanty urination**,
- **pyuria**, with cloudy, **albuminous**, often foul-smelling urine, which sometimes contains blood.

The overall signs are generally **discreet**: a high body temperature or sharp pain located in the costovertebral angle may indicate an associated kidney infection.

When confronted with an apparent case of cystitis, the practitioner must **ask for cytochemical and bacteriological tests of the urine** which may reveal a significant bacteriuria with albuminuria (more than 10^9 bacteria per liter); otherwise, it is cystitis with clear urine.

In the case of recurrence, the following tests must also be performed:

- an inoculation of guinea pigs,
- an intravenous urography,

to rule out an organic lesion of the urogenital tract: malformation (vesicoureteral reflux), tumor (of the kidney, bladder, or prostate), lithiasis, tuberculosis.

Before we study the principal homeopathic medicines for acute cystitis, it has to be said that conventional antibacterial treatment often gives faster results in the case of an isolated attack. On the other hand, homeopathic therapy is preferable for **the treatment of acute episodes of the chronic disease**; it is also preferable for the constitutional treatment of this chronic urinary infection (*Homeopathic Therapeutics: Possibilities in chronic pathology*) ; the earlier the treatment is started, the more effective it is.

Cantharis

This remedy is indicated for cystitis accompanied by **sharp burning pain before, during, and after urination**.

Urination is frequent and **scanty**. The male or female patient may feel concomitant sexual excitement to some degree. The urine is dark and sometimes bloody.

Prescribe in 9 or 15C, five pellets every hour or every two hours depending on the severity of the case; increase the interval with improvement. It is often useful to alternate *Cantharis* with:

Mercurius corrosivus

The clinical signs of this remedy are even more intense than with *Cantharis*. **Hyperalgesic tenesmus** is the dominant feature. Urine is scanty, dark, or markedly bloody.

Prescribe in 9C, five pellets every hour or every two hours, alternately with *Cantharis*. Increase interval between doses with improvement.

Arsenicum album

The pain is **excessively burning**, relieved by applying heat. **But the main sign** is that it has a **marked general effect**. The patient is pale and weak; he goes through alternate periods of anxious agitation and prostration; he is thirsty for frequent small amounts of cold water.

Prescribe in 9C every two to three hours. Increase interval with improvement.

Terebinthina

This remedy is indicated by the particular aspect of the urine: **hematuria with black or dark blood,** which makes up a deposit resembling coffee grounds with an aromatic odor, traditionally compared with the odor of violets.

Prescribe in 5C, five pellets four times a day.

Staphysagria

This remedy is more specially indicated for "traumatic" cystitis in young brides, alternately with *Cantharis* or *Mercurius solubilis*, depending on the symptoms. The remedy is also very useful for **cystalgia after catheterization.**

Prescribe in 9C, five pellets twice a day.

Anticolibacillary serum

Whichever germ is involved, this medicine is **systematically** associated with the above-mentioned remedy or remedies which are indicated by the patient's reactive mode.

Prescribe in 3X, one ampule before each of the three meals, in a very small quantity of pure water, to be kept in the mouth for a moment before swallowing.

EXAMPLE OF PRESCRIPTION FOR ACUTE CYSTITIS

1. Before each of the three meals, an ampule in a very small quantity of non-sparkling mineral water of
   Anticolibacillary serum 3X (n°24)
2. In-between meals, alternate every hour five pellets of
   Cantharis 9C (2 multi-dose tubes)

with five pellets of
   Mercurius corrosivus 9C (2 multi-dose tubes)

Increase interval between doses with improvement. Lots of liquids.

RENAL COLIC

This is a painful, violent attack in the lumbar region, generally spreading toward the lower abdomen and the thighs, often accompanied by paralytic functional ileus and vomiting; the attacks are related to a recent obstacle, ureteral lithiasis being the most frequent but not the exclusive cause.

We will only talk here about the passage of urinary stones in the ureters.

The patient suffering from this hyperalgesic syndrome wants rapid relief. But the pain is so intense that he is not always able to analyze his symptoms in a very precise manner, which may hamper the definition of the homeopathic semiology. Administering conventional antispasmodics is therefore often justified, with the addition of homeopathically indicated remedies. One of these should be prescribed **systematically**:

Calcarea carbonica

This remedy may sometimes be sufficient in itself to relieve the pain and help the elimination of the stone. The prescription is determined by the **physiopathologic similarity**; as Pr. Jean Hamburger emphasized, it is important to consider "**the role of cation in the genesis of lithiasic precipitates**. Lithiasis is always referred to as being phosphatic, oxalic, etc.; in fact, it is made of calcium phosphate, calcium oxalate (much more infrequently, magnesium), and **calcium probably plays a much more important role than acid ions in the mechanism of crystallization**. Such a notion is more particularly based on the observation of hyperparathyroidism lithiasis and so-called immobilization lithiasis, and, lastly, of calciuria in common lithiasis"[11]. Furthermore, the antispasmodic action of calcium ions is recognized by conventional medicine.

The best dilutions are the 15 or 30C, five pellets **every quarter of an hour**; increase interval with improvement.

Pareira brava

This remedy can also be systematically prescribed because of its specific action on the painful spasms of the urinary organs. The pain is accompanied by a constant desire to urinate, but the patient has to exert himself considerably to eliminate a very small amount of urine (he urinates better in a squatting position).

Prescribe in low dilutions 3 or 6X, twenty drops every quarter of an hour, alternately with *Calcarea carbonica*.

Other remedies may be associated, depending on the patient's symptoms:

(11) Hamburger J., Pasteur-Valéry-Radot, Lhermitte F., *Pathologie Médicale*, tome II, Ed. Flammarion; p.196.

Arnica

This remedy is indicated in the case of **associated hematuria**. Because of its specific action on the capillaries, it reduces hemorrhage, accelerates the resorption of edema or of blood suffusion around the stones.

Prescribe in 9C, five pellets three or four times a day.

Colocynthis

The pain is very violent, **paroxysmal, cramp-like**, and does not give the patient much respite. It is **improved by heat, by strong pressure** on the lumbar or abdominal region, and **by flexion** (the patient lies curled up).

Prescribe in 9 or 15C, five pellets every ten to fifteen minutes. Increase interval with improvement.

Lycopodium

The attack occurs mainly between 4 and 8 p.m.; **it is often located on the right side.** This right lateral dominance is relevant during a renal colic attack, but should not be taken into account in the treatment of the lithiasic constitution (*Homeopathic therapeutics: Possibilities in chronic pathology*).

Prescribe a single unit-dose in 15C.

Berberis vulgaris

The pain is stinging, burning, aggravated by strong pressure. It is mostly felt on the **left side**.

Prescribe in 4 or 5C, five pellets four or five times a day.

Sarsaparilla

The pain is intolerable **at the end of urination** and is sometimes accompanied by **violent tenesmus**. The patient finds it easier to urinate standing up (even if he is confined to bed, he has to get up to urinate).

Prescribe in 6X, twenty drops four or five times a day. Increase interval with improvement.

Belladonna

The throbbing-like paroxysmal pain is aggravated by the slightest touch and by jolting movements. The abdomen and the loins are sensitive to the slightest contact. Very often, there are general signs: fever, cephalic congestion, sensorial hyperesthesia.

In fact, the symptoms indicating this remedy are those of a complicated renal colic which must be watched closely, preferably in a surgical ward, and the remedy is only to be prescribed for a few hours before hospital treatment.

Apis mellifica

This remedy may be indicated because of a superadded ureteral edema.

Prescribe in 9 or 15C, every half-hour.

•••••••••

VOMITING OF PREGNANCY

Vomiting during the first three months of pregnancy is a complaint which is of no consequence, but is uncomfortable for the pregnant woman. In some cases, vomiting is unavoidable, leading to severe dehydration and malnutrition, a picture which requires strict isolation and parenteral feeding in hospital.

Usually, nausea and sickness are frequent, with characteristic modalities: aggravation caused by active or passive movement, aggravation on seeing or smelling food, sialorrhea, spasms of the digestive tract, sensation of fainting.

The disorders stop rapidly with homeopathic treatment, with no side effects for the mother and the fetus. The medicines are chosen from the following pharmacodynamic substances:

Sepia

Whatever their usual reactive mode, most pregnant women display symptoms of the proving of *Sepia* during pregnancy. Indeed, during the first few months there is:

- **a sensation of gastric emptiness** which is not improved with eating;
- **nausea from seeing or smelling food**;
- **morning nausea** before breakfast;
- **aversion to tobacco smoke**;
- **vomiting after meals**;
- **craving for slightly acidic or vinegary food** and condiments;
- heartburn with a bad taste in the mouth.

Prescribe in 9C, five pellets twice a day.

Ipeca

Two elements are dominant in the proving of *Ipeca*:

- **a vagotonic element** with **constant nausea**, pale face, bluish rings around the eyes, bradycardia, arterial hypotension, sweating, digestive hypersecretion;
- **a spasmodic element** with **frequent vomiting** of frothy mucus.

The full meaning of these elements is clarified by the characteristic modalities:

- **vomiting does not relieve the nausea**;
- **the tongue remains clear** or lightly coated, and is very humid due to **sialorrhea**;
- **lack of thirst** is frequently observed;
- the nausea is aggravated by movement.

Prescribe in 9C, in timing with the attacks of nausea.

Colchicum autumnale

The smell of food provokes nausea accompanied by **sialorrhea** and **sensations of fainting**. Vomiting contains a lot of mucus and bile; it is **aggravated by the slightest movement** and the pregnant woman describes a cold sensation in the epigastric fossa.

Eggs and fish are not tolerated.

Prescribe in 5C two or three times a day before meals.

Bryonia alba

Vomiting is often bilious; it is **triggered by movement** and diminishes if the woman remains still. The mouth is dry and there is **intense thirst**. Nausea and sickness occur as soon as the patient gets up.

Cabbage is not tolerated.

Prescribe in 9C, two or three times a day.

Kreosotum

Pyrosis occurs at the end of meals; for quite a long time afterwards, **burning vomiting of non-digested food** occurs.

Prescribe in 5C, five pellets before the meal.

Iris versicolor

Its proving is very similar to that of *Kreosotum;* it is more indicated in the case of concomitant migraine.

Same dosage.

Cocculus indicus

The action during provings depends mainly on its principal alkaloid, **picrotoxin**, a violent poison of the central nervous system, particularly of the eighth cranial nerve, and of the motor fibers of the spinal cord.

This remedy is indicated for nausea and vomiting with a **sensation of violent vertigo and yawning**, sometimes associated with great weariness.

These symptoms are aggravated by visual excitement, strong odors (tobacco), and by lack of sleep. These are **relieved by heat**.

Prescribe in 9C, twice a day.

Tabacum

The clinical picture corresponds to that of the real vagal crisis:

- **paleness** followed by **sialorrhea**, cold sweating;
- **nausea** or **sickness;**
- **palpitations** with vertigo and a feeling of faintness.

There is sometimes concomitant diarrhea with a sensation of cold in the abdomen. The patient feels worse from the slightest movement and heat; **fresh air outside** causes improvement, as does closing the eyes.

Same dosage.

Lobelia inflata

As with *Tabacum*, there is a picture of **real vagal crisis**, but the modalities are different:

- **aggravation in the morning on awakening and at night**;
- **improvement by drinking a little**.

Same dosage.

Ignatia amara

This is a remedy for **spasms and paradoxical modalities**; it is useful with **anxious, hypersensitive women**, who describe sensations of constriction in the area of the neck or the epigastric fossa which are temporarily improved by sighing deeply. **Nausea is improved by eating or with distraction**.

This remedy is mainly prescribed because of behavioral particularities; it gives reliable results in

9C, five pellets once or twice a day (on awakening and at bed time).

Nux vomica

This medicine, which is quite seldom used for nausea during pregnancy, is justified when the nausea occurs after meals, there is gastric **intolerance to coffee**, and when the general signs of the remedy are also present (in particular an irrepressible need for a siesta, nervous hypersensitivity, insomnia in the middle of the night).

Prescribe in 9C before the meals.

DELIVERY AND POSTPARTUM PERIOD

The use of homeopathic remedies, suitably chosen according to their pathogenetic symptoms, makes it possible for the homeopath to:

- **facilitate labor**,
- **prevent immediate complications during delivery**,
- **treat the problems of lactation** and re-establish a good overall condition.

HOMEOPATHIC TREATMENT TO FACILITATE LABOR

In this chapter, we shall not deal with any of the mechanical causes which may hamper a normal labor (narrow pelvis, placenta previa, etc.) except for the difficulties encountered during expulsion due to **dystocia of the cervix**.

For women who are expected to be able to deliver normally, and mainly for primiparous women whose labor is always longer than for multiparous women, the following two medicines can be prescribed almost systematically:

Actaea racemosa

The proving of this remedy shows an affinity for the female sexual organs; it is used for **intense and irregular delivery pains due to spasms of the cervix** which hamper dilatation.

Improvement is effected by bending the knees back onto the pelvis. The pain often spreads towards the hips.

The prescription can be started as a preventive measure a fortnight before the theoretical date of the delivery: five pellets in 7 or 9C, morning and evening. The doses are repeated every half-hour as soon as labor starts, then every quarter of an hour after the rupture of the amniotic membrane.

Caulophyllum

This remedy is used for **very violent, irregular, non-productive**, cramp-like delivery **pains**, which do not "push downwards", because of the stiffness of the uterine cervix.

The pain spreads to the groins, the bladder, and the lower limbs.

Prescribe in 4 or 5C at the same frequency as *Actaea racemosa*. These two remedies are prescribed to be taken alternately during labor.

•••••••••

Towards the end of pregnancy, mainly for primiparous women, there may be some anxiety and fear in anticipation of the delivery. The remedies indicated in the chapter "Nervous Anticipation - Acute Reactive Emotional Disorders" on p. 109 are then indicated. *Ignatia* and *Gelsemium* are most frequently prescribed.

PREVENTIVE TREATMENT FOR IMMEDIATE POSTPARTUM PERIOD

After expulsion of the baby, it is useful to systematically prescribe three medicines whose provings correspond to the reactive symptoms generally observed:

- soreness of the perineal and vulvorectal regions;
- vascular disorders: hemorrhoids, risk of uterine hemorrhage, risk of phlebitis, petechiae of the face appearing in mothers who have greatly exerted themselves during expulsion;
- asthenia;
- reactive, or possibly infectious febrile syndrome.

Arnica montana

This remedy is useful to both prevent and treat:

- **pain and the edematous reaction** resulting from the traumatism of the perineal and vulvorectal regions;
- **the risk of hemorrhage** of the post partum (in the case of declared uterine hemorrhage, see chapter "Hemorrhages", p. 222);
- **acute hemorrhoidal problems** (see p. 228);
- **risk of thrombophlebitis** (see p. 225);
- **painful adynamic febrile syndromes**.

Prescribe five pellets of *Arnica 9C* twice a day.

China rubra

This remedy is for **asthenia, weakness, anemia, and arterial hypotension** following the loss of organic liquids; its homeopathic indication is based on this notion as well as on **bloating** and abdominal **meteorism** with **contact hyperesthesia**.

Prescribe in 9C in the morning on awakening for 10 to 14 days.

Pyrogenium

This nosode is prepared from a septic autolysate of a mixture of beef, pork, and human placenta; it ensures the prevention of **adynamic febrile syndromes** of infectious origin.

Prescribe a unit-dose tube in 9C in the evening before going to bed, for one week for example.

PROBLEMS OF LACTATION

Breast-feeding is preferable to all other forms of feeding where possible, particularly since bottle-feeding seems to encourage allergic reactions in genetically-prone individuals. During breast-feeding several problems may occur:

- **insufficient milk production**;
- **mammary engorgement** which may cause abscess of the breast;
- **fissuring** of the nipples;
- **asthenia during breast-feeding**;
- **persistent galactorrhea** after weaning;
- **transitory alopecia** in a more or less depressive context.

INSUFFICIENT MILK PRODUCTION

Lactation may be encouraged by using the following medicines associated, of course, with an appropriate diet and hydration:

Ricinus communis

Low dilutions increase secretion in **hypogalactia**.

Prescribe five pellets of *Ricinus 5C*, twice a day.

Agnus castus

The chaste tree has been well-known since antiquity for its depressing action on the genital function and the secretion of sexual hormones.

This substance was used for a long time in material doses to help people respect vows of chastity. It also has a depressing action on the psyche.

Consequently, it is used in homeopathic medicine for **agalactia** in mothers of new-born children suffering from a **reactive depressive syndrome**.

Prescribe five pellets of *Agnus castus 5C* twice a day.

ENGORGED BREASTS

When galactorrhea is plentiful, an inflammatory, painful, congestive process can be observed in part of the mammary gland and this is sometimes accompanied by a febrile reaction. A fast regression of these symptoms may be obtained with homeopathic therapy. The use of antibiotics, which could put a stop to breast-feeding because of contamination of the mother's milk, is thereby avoided.

Four medicines will be discussed in this context:

Belladonna

This remedy corresponds to the symptomatic tetrad of inflammation:

- **tumefaction** with a sudden onset (tumor);
- **redness** of the integument with a shiny tight skin (rubor);
- **throbbing pain** (dolor);
- intense, radiating **heat**, with a burning sensation (calor).

There is no clear or characteristic modality of improvement through heat or cold, or of presence or lack of thirst. The only general signs, if present, to be considered are the general hypersensitivity of the patient, cephalic congestion with dejection, profuse sweating which brings relief, and sometimes an increase in body temperature.

Prescribe five pellets of *Belladonna 9C* every hour, then increase the interval between doses as the intensity of the symptoms decrease.

Apis mellifica

This remedy corresponds to a large **inflammatory edema** in a region with loose subcutaneous cellular tissue. The skin is less red and shiny than for *Belladonna*, and even sometimes dull. The edema is **burning, stinging, and improved by applying something cold**. The patient's skin may alternately be sweating and dry; she may be febrile; she does not feel thirsty.

The dosage is the same as for *Belladonna*.

Bryonia alba

The breasts are **engorged, very heavy** and hard to the touch, and are the source of intense **pain aggravated by abrupt movement of the mammary gland.** A tight brassiere is required for walking. The integument is slightly rubescent. If there is a febrile reaction, the body temperature is moderate and accompanied by intense thirst.

Same dosage.

Rana bufo

This is the specific remedy for traces of **localized lymphangitis**.

Prescribe in 5C every three or four hours, then increase interval between doses with improvement.

•••••••••

Local treatment consists of:

- ensuring the milk is extracted with a breast pump; this milk must be discarded;
- applying antiphlogistic plaster locally.

•••••••••

If the patient has an abscess on the breast, follow the same procedure as for suppurative processes in soft tissues. The same local treatment is applied.

•••••••••

FISSURING OF THE NIPPLE

The most important thing is to avoid the development of fissures by using local preventive treatment, which should be started in the month before delivery. To effect a sort of tanning of the nipples, the future mother should apply a mixture of equal parts of 45° alcohol and glycerin to the tips of the breasts twice a day. This should be carried out after each feeding throughout the entire nursing period.

If a fissure appears, glycerinated alcohol should be applied, then some *Pommade Castor Equi*; then cover with a sterile gauze compress. In this case, before each feeding, the nipples should be rinsed with boiled water or with flat mineral water until the ointment has been removed. Additionally, two homeopathic medicines help with the cicatrization of fissures:

Graphites

This remedy is indicated for fissures with **thick, viscous, yellow oozing which resembles honey**. When the discharge dries up, a more or less thick crust with a light to brown yellow color appears. Discharge and small crusts are often both present on the same lesion.

High dilutions are used to dry up this discharge. Prescribe five pellets of *Graphites 15C* morning and evening. Increase interval with improvement.

Nitricum acidum

The characteristic fissure treated with this remedy has **clean edges** as if it had been made by a nail or with a cutting tool. **The center bleeds easily.** There is a **stinging sensation**, as if a thorn or splinter was present.

Prescribe in 9C, five pellets two or three times a day. Increase interval with improvement.

ASTHENIA DURING NURSING

This type of asthenia can be fairly rapidly corrected by using one or more remedies to be chosen from:

China rubra

This is the remedy for weakness, anemia, and asthenia after a **significant loss of organic fluid**.

Prescribe five pellets in 9C, twice a day for a month.

Silicea

This remedy for asthenia, weight loss, and demineralization has a clear indication, which is **backache during breast-feeding**. The young woman may also display excessive sensitivity to cold as well as profuse sweating, mainly in the feet.

Prescribe five pellets twice a day or a daily unit-dose tube in 9C for a month.

Demineralization may be treated in the following manner:

Calcarea phosphorica

This medicine is prescribed for long-limbed women who tend to be thin and who display the following phenotype:

- dolichocephalia;
- rectangular teeth with a large vertical axis;
- long hands with fingers which are longer than the palm;
- relative laxity of ligaments;
- tendency towards kyphosis or dorsal scoliokyphosis.

Same dosage as *Silicea*.

Avena sativa and Alfalfa

These two medicines, when used in low dilutions, stimulate the appetite and have an overall invigorating action.

Prescribe twenty drops of the following mixture, to be taken at midday and in the evening before the meal:

Avena sativa 3X
Alfalfa 3X } ana, q.s. to 30 ml

diluted in a little pure water.

PERSISTENCE OF GALACTORRHEA AFTER WEANING

Once lactation has started, it is maintained by the sucking of the nipples if there is sufficient hydration. During weaning, the diminishing frequency of the feedings, accompanied by a relative dehydration caused by taking mild diuretics, should theoretically cause the secretion of milk to dry up. However, women with persistent galactorrhea should use:

Ricinus communis

This medicine has already been cited for promoting lactation when used in low dilutions. Here, it is used in high dilutions to obtain the opposite effect.

Prescribe five pellets of *Ricinus 30C* twice a day until the secretion stops.

RELATIVE TRANSITORY ALOPECIA

Very often, there is hair loss to a greater or lesser extent during the first weeks following delivery. This reason for consulting is very often accompanied by a familiar, more or less discreet, reactive anxiety and depression syndrome.

It is possible to solve this problem with homeopathic therapy using constitutional treatment which includes constitutional as well as symptomatic remedies (*Homeopathic therapeutics: Possibilities in chronic pathology*). As far as transitory alopecia is concerned, hair grows back faster when the following remedy is prescribed together with constitutional treatment:

Eberthinum or Paratyphoidinum B

Typhoid fever is well-known for provoking abundant loss of hair at the end of the progression of the disease.

These nosodes which are prepared from antiseptic-free lysates of Salmonella typhi and paratyphi B cultures are recommended here in 15C, one dose every week or every other week.

CHAPTER VI

SKIN AND MUCOUS MEMBRANES

CUTANEOUS
BURNS

Burns refers to the full range of lesions due to heat. There are three degrees of severity involved:

- **first-degree burns**: simple painful erythema;
- **second-degree burns**: delimited bullae or large phlyctenular bulges on a red and edematous surface; deep second-degree burns: same aspect, but the entire epidermis is affected, including the malpighian layer;
- **third-degree burns**: the integument and subjacent tissues are carbonized.

The severity of the burn depends not only on its degree but on the extent of the lesions. Homeopathy acts effectively on localized burns, diminishing pain and accelerating cicatrization. Extensive burns must obviously be treated in hospital, but they may be improved by the additional use of our remedies.

FIRST-DEGREE BURNS

This erythematous burn is observed, for example, after exposure to the sun or after having been too close to a source of heat.

Belladonna

This remedy is indicated for two specific types of cutaneous aspect:

- either for a **scarlet-red fine eruption**, like that of scarlet fever, **on a dry, mat skin**;
- or a **red, shiny, inflammatory erythematous and edematous eruption, which radiates heat**.

There is a throbbing pain, aggravated by touch, but there is no well-defined thermal modality.

Prescribe five pellets in 5C to be taken every hour or every two hours depending on the severity of the symptoms.

Apis mellifica

This remedy is suitable for **burning, erythematous and edematous eruptions which sting** like a multitude of red hot needles . The skin is reddish pink, rather mat or not very shiny, with sometimes the aspect of orange peel. **The pain is relieved by applying something cold**.

Prescribe five pellets in 9C every hour or every two hours, increasing the interval between doses with improvement.

Local care of erythematous burns is kept to a minimum. Avoid non-penetrating greasy substances which make up real occlusive dressings. It is better to spray pure water or a slightly alcoholic lotion on the burn.

SECOND-DEGREE BURNS

They are generally encountered either after severe sunburn, or after burns from boiling liquids. Their characteristic is the formation of more or less extensive phlyctenae which all respond to:

Cantharis

This remedy is used for **large phlyctenoid vesicles** which contain a clear liquid at the beginning, with subjacent edema. Sometimes there are associated urinary phenomena of the oliguria type.

Prescribe five pellets in 9C four times a day, if necessary alternating with *Apis 9C* in the case of mixed edematous and phlyctenoid lesions. In extensive burns, the patients may display associated urinary phenomena: oliguria, albuminuria, hematuria, cylindruria. At this stage they require hospital care in specialized wards, but in addition, they may usefully benefit from the same homeopathic therapy, since the remedies *Apis* and *Cantharis* display exactly the same urinary phenomena described above in their respective provings.

Locally, and to avoid superinfection, paint the lesions with:

eosin	2 g,
30% alcohol	q.s. to 100 ml.

If the lesions are found on the mucous membranes or near them, use only an aqueous eosin solution of the same concentration.

Extensive phlyctenae must be covered with sterile dressings after aseptic puncture. Tulle gras is extremely useful in such cases.

THIRD-DEGREE BURNS

These are ulcerative burns with necrosis of the living tissue which are generally the consequence of more or less prolonged contact with the source of heat. Three principal remedies may help with the cicatrization of these destructive lesions.

Kali bichromicum

This remedy is suitable for **ulcerations with clear edges** which look as if they had been punched and which are not painful or are barely painful. **The center of the eschar is greenish-yellow** and exudes thick, thready mucus which is not easily detached from the damaged tissues.

Prescribe in 5C, five pellets four times a day.

Arsenicum album

Indicated in the case of **burning pain** with recrudescence at night, relieved by the local application of heat. The serous fluid is excoriating, sanious, and sometimes nauseating. The general condition is affected and there is asthenia and anxious agitation.

Prescribe five pellets in 9C two to four times a day.

Kreosotum

This remedy has practically the same local symptoms as *Arsenicum album*, but includes a tendency towards hemorrhaging and no aggravation at night.

Prescribe five pellets in 5 C four times a day.

•••••••••

Whatever remedy is chosen, it may be associated with *Pyrogenium 9C*, five pellets once or twice a day, to avoid infectious complications.

Locally, wash the healthy peripheral skin with soap and wash the lesions with diluted *Calendula MT*, then paint the skin around the wound with an eosin solution and make a dressing using *Calendula Ointment*. The formula with *Pommade Calendula par digestion* gives excellent results, as proven in clinical tests with this product[12].

VICIOUS CICATRICES

Homeopathic treatment generally gives good results for burns, leaving supple, painless, scarcely visible scars.

However, in subjects who have not been treated, or in patients with a predisposition to keloids, scars with a characteristic fibrous roll can be observed. Homeopathy is certainly the only therapeutic method which can offer treatment for keloid scars that is at the same time preventive and curative, as well as effective and non-aggressive. Curative treatment however is effective only for recent keloids (less than three or four months old).

Graphites

This is the standard symptomatic remedy for **keloid scars**.

Prescribe five pellets in 9C twice a day for one or two months. As a curative measure it is sometimes useful to resort to the 15C dilution. Every evening make an occlusive dressing and apply *Pommade Graphites* locally; the sole inconvenience of *Pommade Graphites* is that it is very messy.

The prescription of *Graphites* is reinforced by that of a weekly dose of *Thuja 15* or *30C*. *Thuja* is the principal remedy of a particular reactive constitution, one of the fundamental characteristics of which is to produce constructive lesions of the skin.

Causticum

This remedy may be useful for painful **vicious cicatrices**, with a fine, fragile, unhealthy skin which feels like an raw, open graze.

Prescribe five pellets in 5C twice a day.

•••••••••

(12) Dr. Marduel, *5th Congress of the Société Française d'Etude et de Traitement des Brûlés*, Lyon, 21st september 1984.

ACUTE URTICARIA

Urticarial rash is characterized by a collection of **serous papules** which are red or pinkish and sometimes faded in the center, similar to nettle stings. They are the result of the **local release of histamine** due to the effect of a conflict between antigen and antibody, which causes papillary edema with **pruritus and a sensation of burning**.

This rash, which appears suddenly, is temporary. It generally disappears after a few hours or a few days, leaving no traces. It may remain local, or, on the contrary, spread out, accompanied by spectacular edema, specially around the eyelids. In this case, we refer to giant urticaria or Quincke's edema whose seriousness is due to concomitant edema in the larynx. We will not study this severe and localized form as it is generally treated by conventional means. Homeopathy, however, may be a useful adjuvant in acute attacks. It is essential in the constitutional treatment of recurrent forms.

MEASURES TO BE TAKEN

In the case of recent urticaria of sudden onset the triggering cause or allergen must be investigated:

- **triggering contact**: nettles, thuja, insects, etc.;
- **triggering cause**: mainly cold, heat, sun, exertion, emotional stress, etc.;
- **food** which is known for being liable to cause urticaria attacks: strawberries, chocolate, shellfish, fish, etc.;
- **triggering medicine**: aspirin, barbiturate, sulfonamide, penicillin, vaccine, serum, etc.

In cases of recurrent urticaria, a microbial, parasitic, mycotic, or endocrine origin, malignant lymphoma, neoplasia, etc. should be looked for.

The homeopathic practitioner must, as always, make a precise nosologic diagnosis.

HOMEOPATHIC TREATMENT

Homeopathic treatment uses three groups of remedies, possibly combined, that is to say the medicines are taken separately at a greater or lesser interval between doses depending on the severity of the symptoms:

- **chemical mediators** in infinitesimal dilutions;
- **allersodes prepared from the allergen**;
- **remedies based on the phenomenon of similars**.

Results are generally good and fast.

CHEMICAL MEDIATORS

Histaminum

Histamine is one of the chemical mediators of allergic reactions. The *in vitro* action of *Histaminum 7C* on basophil degranulation from allergic patients is well-known.

Prescribe *Histaminum 7C*, five pellets every hour or every two hours, increasing the interval between doses with improvement.

Lung histamine

This sarcode is prepared from the lungs of a guinea-pig which has been sacrificed in a state of anaphylactic shock; it contains histamine as well as many other chemical mediators: bradykinin, serotonin, PAF-acether, etc.

It has been clinically used in 9 or 15C for decades and has often proved to be effective.

There are no clinical criteria, other than therapeutic trials on the same patient, on which to base a choice between *Histaminum* and *Lung Histamine*.

ALLERSODES PREPARED FROM THE ALLERGEN

This technique is only possible when the allergen is known since it consists in giving the patient hahnemannian dilutions prepared from his own allergen (*Homeopathic Therapeutics: Possibilities in chronic pathology*, p. 65).

This process can only be used for recurrent urticaria. In this case, the remedy can be prepared in advance and possibly given as a preventive measure.

It is prescribed in 15C, five pellets once or twice a day. It should be emphasized that these cases are paroxysmal episodes of a particular chronic constitution.

REMEDIES ACCORDING TO THE PHENOMENON OF SIMILARS

Apis mellifica

This remedy is indicated when the skin is reddish pink and sometimes infiltrated like orange peel. When the subcutaneous cellular tissue is looser, it has a more marked edematous and red aspect, for example around the eyelids.

In every case the skin stings and burns as if it was being stung by a multitude of red hot needles. It is **relieved by applying something cold** and aggravated by heat. Pruritus has the same modalities.

This remedy has a **rapid but short-lasting action**. Prescribe *Apis 9* or *15C*, five pellets every thirty minutes. Increase interval with improvement.

Urtica urens

This remedy is indicated for stinging and burning edema which is paler than the edema of *Apis* and causes unbearable pruritus. The symptoms are **aggravated by applying something cold**, taking a bath, washing, **and above all by touch**.

Prescribe five pellets in 5C two to four times a day, increasing the interval with improvement.

Sulphur

This major remedy is indicated in the case of a pruritic and burning eruption in a fairly sthenic subject with a tendency towards periodical cutaneous, mucous, or serous complaints. These complaints may alternate with each other or with internal symptoms: liver, hemorrhoids, and high blood pressure.

Urticaria is aggravated by heat, water, and relieved by cold.

Prescribe a single dose in 15C, in association with *Apis* or *Urtica urens*.

Psorinum

This nosode may be indicated in two specific cases:

- either for a patient who is **generally asthenic and sensitive to cold** and who displays an alternating overall pathological condition of the same type as *Sulphur*,
- or for a patient **who does not react at all or does not react well** to *Sulphur*.

Prescribe a single dose in the first case, and *Psorinum* in a scaled dosage (*9-12-15-30C*, one dose a day on four following days) in the second case.

•••••••••

INSECT BITES

Insect bites (bees, wasps, mosquitoes, spiders, etc.) may cause painful local reactions with edema and inflammation. In particularly sensitive subjects these reactions may become general or lead to complications with allergic phenomena.

In the majority of cases patients are relieved by one or more of the following remedies chosen according to their specific reactive features.

Apis mellifica

This remedy is almost always indicated. It corresponds to bites followed by the sudden appearance of **pinkish edema** with **burning, stinging pain which is relieved by applying something cold.**

Prescribe five pellets in 9C every quarter of an hour, increasing the interval with improvement.

Tarentula cubensis

This remedy is indicated when the bite causes inflammation with **localized, painful induration** accompanied by a sensation of intense burning. During the following days it may become **bluish and ecchymotic** and sometimes lead to satellite adenopathy.

Prescribe in 9C, two to four times a day depending on the severity of the symptoms.

Cantharis

This remedy is suitable when the bite causes a **phlyctenoid reaction** with large, burning, pruritic vesicles which are improved by applying something cold.

Prescribe in 9C, two to four times a day, increasing the interval with improvement which generally takes two to three days.

Ledum palustre

This remedy may be indicated in the case of papular, pruritic, painful lesions, with a local feeling of coldness, relieved by applying something cold.

But the most interesting thing about it is that, if taken morning and evening for example, it curiously seems to prevent people who are constitutionally more vulnerable than average from being bitten.

Prescribe in 5C, morning and evening, throughout the stay in the infested area.

If the bites show the initial signs of superinfection, prescribe five pellets of *Pyrogenium 9C* morning and evening as well as the chosen treatment, and, in the case of **lymphangitis**, *Rana bufo 5C* every six hours approximately.

Apply a cotton wool pad soaked in the following mixture to the sting:

Calendula MT }
Ledum palustre MT } ana, q.s. to 30 ml

For patients who display severe allergic reactions to insect bites, a specific constitutional treatment has to be considered, since the reaction is in fact an acute manifestation (often requiring conventional remedies) of a specific chronic constitution which can nearly always be improved by homeopathic treatment.

• • • • • • • • • •

apis mellifica — pinkish edema — pain, burning, stinging

tarentula — localized inflam, bluish & ecchymotic — painful, induration, intense burning

cantharis — bullous, phlyctenoid [illegible] — pruritic, burning

ledum palustre — papular — pruritic, painful — feeling of coldness

all improved by cold

ledum palustre used prophylactically in those constitutionally vulnerable to be bitten
5C q am + q pm while stay in infested area

if super infection add
pyrogenium 9C q am & pm

Lymphangitis
Rana bufo 5C q 6 hr

ACUTE NON-ALLERGIC CONJUNCTIVITIS

In this complaint there is **inflammation of the conjunctiva**; the clinical signs are a sensation of the presence of a foreign body, a burning sensation, photophobia, and lacrimation. The conjunctiva is red and hyperemic. There are secretions which are watery at first, then mucous, and may become mucopurulent with its development.

The etiologic diagnosis should be as precise as possible: virus, bacteria, physical agents, conjunctivitis which is symptomatic of a more general complaint (e.g. measles). If necessary, the patient should be examined by an ophthalmologist to make sure the cornea is not affected or that there is no other ocular complaint (glaucoma, etc.).

From the homeopathic point of view, we differentiate the remedies:

- for the onset,
- for catarrhal conjunctivitis,
- for mucopurulent conjunctivitis.

REMEDIES FOR THE ONSET

Aconitum

Conjunctival inflammation appears suddenly, generally after a **sudden chill**; there is **photophobia**.

Prescribe five pellets in 9C every hour, increasing the interval with improvement.

Belladonna

Conjunctivitis with a sudden onset, marked photophobia, intense and sometimes **throbbing pain, local warmth** with a burning sensation, **aggravated by cold air**. The conjunctival mucous membrane remains dry.

Prescribe five pellets in 9C every hour; increase interval with improvement.

Apis mellifica

The conjunctivitis is accompanied by **edema** which appears later, with pruritus, and a stinging, burning pain which is **relieved by applying something cold** and aggravated by heat.

Prescribe in 15C every hour; increase interval with improvement.

REMEDIES FOR CATARRHAL CONJUNCTIVITIS

Euphrasia

Inflamed redness of the conjunctiva with a **burning sensation in the eyes** and the **impression of a foreign body present**.

Abundant flow of irritant, excoriating tears. Swelling and agglutination of the free edge of the eyelids with inflammation and, possibly, ulceration of the conjunctival cul-de-sac.

Aggravation in a warm room and in light.

Prescribe five pellets in 5C every hour; increase interval with improvement.

REMEDIES FOR MUCOPURULENT CONJUNCTIVITIS

Argentum nitricum

Mucopurulent flow sometimes with swollen caruncles. The eyelids may be swollen. Intense photophobia. **Stinging, splinter-like pain**. Aggravation with heat and **improvement with cool air in the open**.

Prescribe five pellets in 9C two to four times a day; increase interval with improvement.

Mercurius solubilis

There is a greenish-yellow, **irritant, corrosive discharge**. The pain is aggravated by heat and light.

The patient also shows the general signs of the remedy: sweating at night, shivering on the surface of the skin, sometimes buccopharyngeal signs.

Prescribe five pellets in 9C two to four times a day.

Pulsatilla

The discharge is yellow or greenish-yellow, creamy, and **in general non-irritant** (the tears may cause irritation).

The symptoms are aggravated in a warm room and improved by fresh air.

Prescribe five pellets in 9C two to four times a day.

Hepar sulphur

This major homeopathic remedy for acute suppuration is indicated for conjunctivitis with a copious, purulent discharge.

Pain is **aggravated by cold, touch**, the slightest draft and **relieved by heat**.

Prescribe one dose in 15 or 30C morning and evening, preceded two hours earlier by five pellets of *Pyrogenium 9C*.

•••••••••

Homeopathic treatment may be active when used alone in a certain number of cases. Otherwise it is a temporary measure while awaiting the results of complementary biological tests, e.g. antibiotic sensitivity test, which will help specify the necessary etiologic treatment.

It is complemented by local care which should be as gentle as possible, for example physiologic salt solution or, even better, borated or non-borated solution which is isotonic with tears.

•••••••••

HERPES ZOSTER

This infectious disease, whose symptom is an eruption of large flaccid vesicles with a unilateral, radicular topography, is caused by the varicella-zoster virus. The eruption is accompanied by adenopathy and neuralgic sensory disorders; it often leaves painful sequelae. It is thought that chicken pox might be the primary viral infection and herpes zoster an exogenous or endogenous reinfection.

The onset period is short, lasting only three or four days. It is characterized by moderate fever, a sick feeling, and pain in the area where the eruption will appear.

The fully-declared phase is characterized by an erythematous and vesicular eruption accompanied by pain with a unilateral, radicular topography. The eruption develops in three phases:

- **an erythematous phase**, with eruptive plaques of a pink, then a red color, rounded or oval in shape;
- **a vesicular phase** (around the 24th hour): the vesicles appear on the eruptive plaques; they are filled with a clear liquid and are first grouped in clusters, then converge in bullae.
- **a desiccation phase** (around the 5th or 7th day): the vesicles become cloudy and are covered with a yellowish crust.

The eruption is accompanied by a discreet infectious syndrome, satellite adenopathy, and above all pain, the intensity of which is unrelated to the extent of the lesions, with disorders of sensitivity in the affected area.

The clinical forms are varied, since all the radicular areas may be affected. However, the most frequent types are thoracic herpes zoster (50% of the cases) and herpes zoster affecting the cranial nerves (15% of the cases), in particular herpes zoster ophthalmicus (5th) and herpes zoster auricularis (7th).

Complications consist essentially of possible phenomena of **superinfection**, but there is above all **postherpetic algesia** which is most frequently observed in elderly subjects. **Paralysis** is more rarely observed.

Homeopathy makes it possible to treat this disease effectively by shortening its progression and avoiding residual pain.

ONSET PHASE

In this phase, the following two remedies should be prescribed systematically:

Staphylococcinum

The promising results obtained in the treatment of herpes zoster by staphylococcic vaccinotherapy have led François Lamasson to administer successfully dilutions of *Staphylococcinum* (a nosode prepared from the pure lysate culture of Staphylococcus pyogenes aureus).

The development of the disease is shortened by prescribing from the onset one dose of *Staphylococcinum 15* or *30C*, repeated on the next three days. The first dose is followed about six hours later by:

Sulphur

This is a remedy with a centrifugal action, which helps all cutaneous eruptions. In doing so, it diminishes the risk of postherpetic neuralgia while revealing more clearly the clinical aspect of the eruption.

Prescribe a single unit-dose tube in 15C.

FULLY-DECLARED PHASE

When the eruption is declared, the **aspect of the cutaneous lesion and its modalities** determine the choice of the remedy.

ERYTHEMATOUS PHASE

Apis mellifica

Remedy for **erythematous eruptions with stinging, burning edema relieved by applying something cold**. The patient is usually not thirsty.

Arsenicum album

This remedy is very often indicated in the treatment of herpes zoster; it corresponds to erythematous and also vesicular eruptions **which burn like embers and are relieved by applying something warm**.

The pain has a nocturnal recrudescence between 1 and 3 a.m. The patient is often worried, agitated, anxious, and thinks he is severely ill indeed because his illness has made him **very weak**. He is thirsty for small, frequently repeated amounts of cold water.

VESICULAR PHASE

Rhus toxicodendron

This remedy is for **small vesicles** of about one millimeter in diameter. They contain **clear, citrine liquid** and sit on a **burning, pruritic, erythematous base**. The pruritus is not relieved by scratching but by continually changing position (hence a certain degree of agitation shown by the patient) and **by applying compresses or taking warm showers**.

Rhus vernix or Rhus venenata

This remedy is used for **small vesicles** which are sometimes more numerous and pruritic than those of *Rhus toxicodendron* but do not have the same characteristic modalities.

Ranunculus bulbosus

This remedy is suitable for **bluish vesicles which contain hematic liquid**. They are very pruritic and cause intense pain, which occurs in paroxysms like being stabbed with a knife. Aggravation with touch or movement.

Localization in the left intercostal spaces is characteristic but is not necessary for the remedy to be prescribed. The blackish-blue, hematic aspect of the vesicles clearly indicates this medicine.

Ranunculus sceleratus

This remedy is more difficult to individualize and so is more rarely prescribed. It corresponds to vesicles containing a yellowish, irritant, serous liquid which causes **sensations of biting**, shooting pain, and **tearing**.

Cantharis

This remedy is frequently indicated and corresponds to **large phlyctenoid vesicles, like bullae**. They are pruritic and burning, improved by coolness or by applying something cold. The concomitance of urinary phenomena has often been described in texts but is rare and is not necessary for the prescription of the remedy. Here again, the prescription is determined by the anatomicopathological aspect of the cutaneous lesion which resembles second-degree burns.

VESICULOUS AND/OR CRUSTED PHASE

Mezereum

This remedy is suitable for two specific cutaneous aspects:

- either burning, pruriginous **vesicles** which contain a **thick, opalescent, white or yellowish liquid**;
- or hard, whitish or brownish, **thick crusts** which, when pressed, exude **whitish or yellowish pus** produced by a small, subjacent ulceration.

This medicine is also suitable for **intercostal or facial neuralgia**, aggravated by touch, movement, by the warmth of the bed at night, but, curiously, relieved by radiating heat.

Prunus spinosa

This remedy is indicated for herpes zoster localized on the **branches of the trigeminal nerve** (herpes zoster ophthalmicus in particular). It corresponds to ocular pain with a bursting sensation in the eyeball, aggravated by contact, accompanied or not by ocular or periocular edema.

Anagallis arvensis

This is a rarely indicated remedy. It corresponds to pruritic vesicles which, when excoriated, become covered with an epidermal film which allows a new vesicle to be formed.

DOSAGE

All these remedies are indicated for cutaneous and/or nervous disorders (tissue of ectodermal origin). High dilutions are generally the most reliable and effective. Therefore, depending on similarity, the 7 or 9C dilution is used if the homeopathic similarity is situated at the level of the cutaneous lesions, and the 15C dilution is used if the homeopathic similarity includes the characteristic modalities of neuralgic processes.

Prescribe five pellets every three or four hours (or depending on the climax of the painful paroxysms). Then increase the interval between doses with improvement.

It is preferable to avoid applying powders and especially ointments locally as they might help maceration of the lesions. On the other hand, to avoid cutaneous superinfection, it is useful to prescribe painting with an antiseptic solution of 2% eosin in 60° alcohol for example.

EXAMPLE OF PRESCRIPTION FOR HERPES ZOSTER OPHTHALMICUS

In this example, the patient displays an edematous and vesicular eruption in the area of the ophthalmic branch of the trigeminal nerve. The pain is intense, burning, stinging, and relieved by cold, and spreads to the eyeball giving an impression of bursting. The eyelids are red and edematous. Prescribe the following:

1. Take a unit-dose tube of

   Staphylococcinum 15C

as soon as possible and let it dissolve in the mouth; six hours later, take a unit-dose tube of

   Sulphur 15C (a single dose).

2. Then approximately every two hours alternate five pellets of

   Apis 9C (2 multi-dose tubes of pellets)
   and *Prunus spinosa 15C* (2 multi-dose tubes of pellets)

and also, on the first two mornings, a unit-dose tube of

   Staphylococcinum 15C (3 doses altogether).

Increase the interval between the doses of *Apis* and *Prunus spinosa* with improvement.

TREATMENT OF COMPLICATIONS

There are three types of complications, as already seen: superinfection of the cutaneous lesions, postherpetic algesia, and paralysis.

SUPERINFECTION

Mezereum

This remedy is sometimes indicated during the fully-declared phase; it is always indicated in the case of cutaneous superinfection which resembles impetiginous lesions: thick crusts covering irritant yellowish pus.

It should almost always be associated with remedies for suppuration:

Pyrogenium

To be prescribed systematically in 9C on awakening and on going to bed with

Hepar sulphur

This remedy is specific for acute suppuration (see chapter "Abscesses and Acute Suppurative Processes", page 93). The affected areas are **hypersensitive to touch** and local pain is **relieved by heat**.

High dilutions are mainly used (15 or 30C) as they slow down suppuration: for example, five pellets morning and evening after taking *Pyrogenium*.

POSTHERPETIC ALGESIA

Postherpetic algesia is exceptional in herpes zoster which has been correctly treated with homeopathy; it is more frequent in elderly subjects. The treatment is all the more difficult if the neuralgia has been present for a long time and has been treated in various ways (corticoids, anti-inflammatory drugs, radiotherapy, etc.).

The remedies which were studied for the fully-declared phase may be indicated if the patient's reactive modes correspond to the modalities of their provings. Most often, *Apis, Arsenicum album, Ranunculus bulbosus, Mezereum* are involved. In addition, the following remedies are necessary:

Hypericum perforatum

This remedy is suitable for pain spreading **along the nerve paths** which is aggravated by jolts or movements.

Prescribe in 15 or 30C, five pellets two to four times a day depending on the severity of the case, or during painful paroxysms.

Kalmia latifolia

This remedy is indicated in the presence of **lightning pain like electric shocks** followed by numbing, aggravated by movement. It is particularly indicated in neuralgia in the face, the right orbit and eye (left side: *Spigelia*).

Prescribe in 15C, five pellets depending on the frequency of the painful paroxysms.

Magnesia phosphorica

This is the remedy for **sporadic, sudden,** cramp-like, erratic, **unbearable pain** which makes the patient cry out, **with a sudden onset and end. Relieved by heat** or by leaning forward.

There is right lateral dominance, particularly for facial or orbital neuralgia, but it is not exclusive.

Prescribe in 15C, five pellets depending on the frequency of the painful paroxysms.

Causticum

This remedy is suitable for neuralgia with **a sensation of scraping** and burning, **as if the skin was raw**. Aggravation with intense, dry cold, or at around three in the morning. **Improvement with rainy, humid and warm weather**. It is also a remedy for residual paralysis mainly located in the face, with ptosis of the eyelid, accompanied by spreading pain.

Prescribe in 15C two to four times a day, depending on the severity of the symptoms.

Vaccinotoxinum

This nosode, which is prepared from smallpox vaccine, is recommended by some authors because of

- the similarity between the eruptive elements of smallpox and those of herpes zoster, on the one hand,
- and the relationship between the viruses responsible, on the other hand.

Prescribe in 15C, five pellets twice a day, then once a day.

Thuja occidentalis

This remedy is particularly beneficial for postherpetic algesia of herpes zoster which has been treated in various ways. It is the principal medicine of "sycosis", a specific reactive mode and a permanent morbid disposition which has been acquired after long drawn-out infections, repeated vaccinations, and intensive antibiotic or corticoid treatments (*Homeopathic Therapeutics: Possibilities in chronic pathology*, p.31). Its proving includes, besides vesicular eruptions, chronic neuralgia.

Prescribe in 15 or 30C, either in weekly doses, or in daily pellets, depending on the clinical cases.

• • • • • • • • •

To summarize, it can schematically be said that, given the patients' habitual reactive modes, postherpetic algesia in general requires *Apis - Arsenicum album - Hypericum - Mezereum - Thuja.*

Residual algesia of herpes zoster ophthalmicus more often requires the prescription of *Prunus spinosa - Kalmia latifolia - Apis - Causticum.*

Algesia consecutive to herpes facialis often indicates: *Magnesia phosphorica* (pain on the right side), *Spigelia* (pain on the left side), and intercostal herpes zoster indicates: *Rhus toxicodendron - Mezereum - Ranunculus bulbosus.*

• • • • • • • • • • • •

PARALYSIS

It is not very frequent and generally regresses in a few weeks. Two remedies have a preferential indication:

Arsenicum album

This remedy is mainly suitable for paralysis of the extremities of the limbs; the paralysis is often preceded or accompanied by contracture and tremor. Burning pain relieved by heat may also be reported, as well as the general signs of the remedy especially with pronounced asthenia.

Prescribe according to similarity in 9, 15, or 30C twice a day.

Causticum

For this remedy the paralysis is more focused and affects mainly the right side. It is a frequent remedy for facial paralysis affecting the eyelids or tongue. There is often tearing, paroxysmal pain, with sensations of burning and as if the integument was exposed. Relief afforded by humid heat is a modality which is not often encountered; aggravation by intense cold is more frequently found.

Same dosage as previously.

• • • • • • • • •

In resistant cases where these remedies are not sufficiently active, the patient's constitutional remedies should be used. These are defined by taking account of the overall progression of the patient's pathological condition (of his chronic reactive mode), his morphology, the changes in behavior concomitant with his illness, and his sensitive type (*Homeopathic Therapeutics: Possibilities in chronic pathology*, p. 37).

• • • • • • • • • • • • • • •

CHAPTER VII

VASCULAR SYSTEM

HEMORRHAGES

Hemorrhages are blood suffusion of varying quantities caused by the breaking of one or more vascular envelopes and possibly involving any organ: soft tissues, bones, mucous membranes and viscera, subsequent to various mechanisms:

- traumatism: an accidental or surgical wound; contusion which may cause ecchymosis, hematoma or effusion, bone fracture, rupture of viscera, hemorrhaging after an abortion;
- complaints involving erosion of the mucous membranes: gastroduodenal ulcer, Crohn's disease, hemorrhagic rectocolitis, hemorrhoids, etc.;
- infectious diseases: nephritis with hematuria, purpura, etc.;
- tumorous processes;
- vascular diseases: rupture of varices, Rendu-Osler-Weber disease, etc.;
- disruption of endocrine secretions: metrorrhagia, metromenorrhagia, etc.;
- disruption of coagulation.

Depending on the case, four problems appear in isolation or in succession:

- **checking the hemorrhage**;
- **correcting the blood volume**;
- **helping the resorption of hematoma and ecchymoses;**
- **facilitating vascular cicatrization** and rapid convalescence.

Once the nosologic diagnosis has been made, different appropriate therapeutic measures must be taken; the contribution of the homeopathic method is far from negligible.

CHECKING THE HEMORRHAGE

Lesions in the large vascular trunks and the rupture of viscera require adequate surgical treatment. As for hemorrhaging involving small vessels, in addition to mechanical compression when possible, the checking of the hemorrhage is facilitated, whatever the etiology, by using the following homeopathic medicines.

Phosphorus

Phosphorus in toxic doses reduces coagulability, leading to **repeated hemorrhages of red blood** which are difficult to control and which may occur in any tissue.

Therefore *Phosphorus 9C* is used, five pellets every half-hour for a few hours for medium-sized hemorrhages, whereas a dose of *Phosphorus 9C* is prescribed every six hours, for example, for hemorrhagic pancreatitis and purpura.

Arnica montana

Its proving disrupts coagulation and shows an affinity for blood vessels, so it is the **standard remedy for venous pathological conditions** and it is used systematically, like *Phosphorus*.

The dosage is identical for medium-sized hemorrhages; all dilutions above the 5C seem to be equally effective. The two remedies are alternated.

Millefolium

This medicine is used for hemorrhages involving **bright red, shiny, fluid blood**. It is principally used for **hemorrhages which spread**: wounds, metrorrhagia of the menopause, etc.

Prescribe *Millefolium* in 5C, five pellets repeated with increased frequency as the symptoms are more pronounced.

Erigeron canadensis

For this choice of remedy, the hemorrhage, generally of gynecological origin, should be **profuse, with bright red, shiny blood**, spurting in successive jets, **aggravated by any movement.**

Its prescription is identical to that of *Millefolium*.

CORRECTING THE BLOOD VOLUME

The only effective treatment in this case is the conventional one.

HELPING THE RESORPTION OF HEMATOMA AND ECCHYMOSES

The earlier the homeopathic treatment is applied, the more effective it is.

Arnica montana

Systematically prescribing *Arnica montana* in any dilution above 5C avoids hemorrhagic suffusion in soft tissues.

Give five pellets every quarter of an hour as soon as possible after the traumatism, then progressively increase the interval between doses.

Ledum palustre

This remedy is used when the **ecchymoses,** which are bluish-red at first, have turned **greenish-yellow**, and take a long time to disappear; a black eye is a typical example.

Prescribe *Ledum palustre 5C*, five pellets four times a day.

FACILITATING VASCULAR CICATRIZATION AND A RAPID CONVALESCENCE

Two remedies should be used systematically: *Arnica* for vascular cicatrization and *China rubra* to facilitate convalescence.

Arnica montana

Prescribe five pellets of *Arnica montana 9C* two to four times a day for the reasons already mentioned.

China rubra

This remedy for **asthenia, weakness, and hypotension** following the loss of organic fluid is indicated in the present case.

Prescribe in 9C, five pellets two to four times a day.

•••••••••

SUPERFICIAL PHLEBITIS OF THE LOWER LIMBS

This complaint used to be incorrectly called periphlebitis. In fact, it is an **inflammation with thrombosis of the varicose veins** with the following symptoms:

- **pain**,
- **redness**,
- **induration** of recent onset.

It causes embolism only in exceptional cases.

The pain remains slight; there is no, or hardly any general effect. It rarely progresses toward thrombosis of the saphena; on the other hand, there is frequent recurrence.

In elderly subjects, subjacent arteriopathy should be investigated.

In the case of very intense perivenous reaction, a thrombogenic cause should be sought: hemopathy, diaphragmatic hernia, digestive or genital cancer, taking of contraceptives, etc.

REMEDIES FOR THE ONSET AND THE FULLY-DECLARED PHASE

Belladonna

For sudden onset of the symptoms, locally accompanied by:

- **redness and tumefaction**,
- **pain**, which is often **throbbing**,
- **intense radiating heat** with a sensation of **burning**.

Prescribe *Belladonna 7C*, five pellets every two hours; increase interval with improvement.

Apis

This remedy is indicated for:

- **pinkish-red edematous inflammation**,
- with **burning, stinging pain**;
- the pain is **improved by applying something cold** and aggravated by heat.

Pruritus with the same modalities may exist.

Prescribe *Apis 9* or *15C*, five pellets every two hours. Increase interval with improvement.

Vipera redi

Experimentation with *Vipera* causes a reaction in the veins of **inflammatory edema** and **lymphangitis**, similar to the reactive mode of superficial phlebitis.

Practically, *Vipera* is therefore indicated for all types of superficial phlebitis when the following signs are found:

- **venous inflammation and dilatation**,
- accompanied by **pain and a sensation of bursting**,
- **aggravated by letting the leg hang down** and relieved by raising it.

Prescribe five pellets of *Vipera 5C* two to four times a day depending on the severity of the symptoms.

Lachesis

This is also a snake venom. Pathogenetic experimentation has revealed an action on the blood with the first phase of hypercoagubility, followed by the second phase of hypocoagulability with ecchymoses.

Lachesis is indicated when the following signs are found:

- **local purplish aspect**, sometimes ecchymotic,
- **a very painful, hyperesthetic vein**,
- **aggravation by heat and touch**.

If superficial phlebitis occurs in a patient whose sensitive type corresponds to that of *Lachesis*, the general symptoms of the remedy may be exacerbated by the local complaint: for example, general hyperesthesia, increased aggressiveness, etc.

Prescribe in 9C, five pellets morning and evening for local similarity; prescribe in 15C when there is exacerbation of the general or behavioral symptoms.

Arnica

The complaint often starts after a direct traumatism or after exertion.

Inflammation may be accompanied by **ecchymosis**. The pain resembles that of **contusion**, myalgia, or muscular pain. It is aggravated by the slightest touch.

In fact, *Arnica*, like *Vipera*, may be systematically prescribed for superficial phlebitis because of its pathogenetic affinity for capillaries.

Prescribe in 9C, five pellets twice a day.

Patients' reactive modes are rarely unequivocal. Therefore, when the symptomatology is polymorphic, it is advisable to give two or three remedies in rotation during the same day. The different remedies then complement each other.

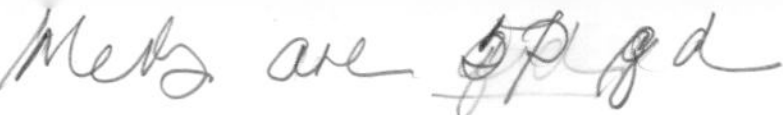

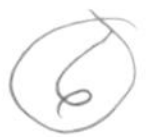

REMEDIES FOR THE PHASE OF RESOLUTION

Remedies with an affinity for the veins should be prescribed for a reasonable length of time to avoid recurrence.

Arnica

For persistent pain, like that caused by contusion or myalgia, which is aggravated by exertion.

Prescribe *Arnica 9C*, five pellets once a day.

Vipera redi

For a sensation of **heavy legs**, quite distinctly **relieved by raising the lower limbs**, and aggravated by letting them hang down.

Prescribe *Vipera 7C*, five pellets once a day.

Hamamelis virginiana

In the case of sensitive and painful, dilated veins, with the sensation of a bruise-type pain, or **of bursting of the veins**. These symptoms are aggravated by heat.

Prescribe *Hamamelis 6X*, fifteen to twenty drops twice a day.

Pulsatilla

In the case of varices with slight throbbing pain, concomitant with **erythrocyanosis of the extremities**. Aggravation by heat and rest. Improvement by walking in the open.

Prescribe *Pulsatilla 7C*, five pellets a day.

Calcarea fluorica

This remedy is indicated when there is persistent **indurated varicose panniculitis**.

Prescribe *Calcarea fluorica* in 9C, five pellets once a day over a long period.

Fluoricum acidum

This remedy is indicated for **pruritic varices**, and/or a **sensation of burning in the legs**.

Aggravation by heat and improvement by coolness.

Same dosage as for *Calcarea fluorica*.

ACUTE HEMORRHOIDAL PROBLEMS

Hemorrhoids are varices in the anus and rectum which are frequently observed when several phenomena are combined in the same patient:

- **portal hypertension**;
- **a constitutional predisposition** which is specific to the subject and associates **venous fragility** and **digestive fragility**.

Acute hemorrhoidal bouts, which are rapidly alleviated by using a symptomatic homeopathic treatment, should be distinguished from recurrent hemorrhoidal development which requires either a constitutional homeopathic treatment or a surgical cure.

These acute hemorrhoidal bouts are encountered in certain precise conditions:

- abuse of alcoholic drinks,
- picture of acute or subacute enteritis consecutive to the ingestion of an excessive amount of spices or pharmacodynamic substances,
- delivery, prolonged exertion, etc.

Under these conditions, inflammation of the hemorrhoidal veins occurs, accompanied by **congestion** which may even lead to **hemorrhaging** or **thrombosis**, sometimes with **pruritus**.

The homeopathic therapy combines an oral treatment with hygiene and dietary care.

REMEDIES FOR VENOUS CONGESTION

Aesculus hippocastanum

In experimental conditions, the horse chestnut tree causes venous plethora with an elective hemorrhoidal effect. The subject has a sensation of **rectal fullness**, of needles in the rectum, and of a **dry, burning,** excoriating **mucous membrane**.

Aesculus hippocastanum 3X or *6X* can be almost systematically prescribed, in a dosage of twenty drops, two to four times a day, diluted in a little pure water, to be kept in the mouth for a moment before swallowing.

Arnica montana

This is the remedy for veins and venous capillaries since *Arnica* has shown an affinity for these tissues during its proving. There is a **sensation of contusion** aggravated by the slightest touch.

Prescribe five pellets of *Arnica 9C* every hour or every two hours. Then increase the interval between the doses as the symptoms diminish in intensity.

Nux vomica

This remedy is indicated to alleviate **very painful hemorrhoids, improved by cold or ice-cold applications**, which appeared after eating too many spices and/or drinking too much alcohol in sthenic, irascible, sedentary subjects who indulge in good food too often and are prone to chronic constipation.

Prescribe five pellets of *Nux vomica 9C* three or four times a day.

Aloe socotrina

This medicine is used for burning hemorrhoids which bulge like a bunch of grapes, with a blue hue, in patients who concomitantly display **sphincteral insecurity** whereby they involuntarily let escape feces or **mucus which is thick like jelly**.

Prescribe in 5C, five pellets twice a day.

Sepia officinalis

This medicine is used as a symptomatic remedy for acute hemorrhoidal bouts when there is **pelvic congestion, constipation, difficult circulation** in the lower limbs, and **painful prolapsed hemorrhoids**. These conditions are often met during pregnancy and delivery.

Prescribe five pellets of *Sepia 7C* two to four times a day.

REMEDIES FOR BLEEDING HEMORRHOIDS

Arnica montana

Naturally, we come across this medicine again, used in the same way as previously mentioned, when, in addition to the sensation of **venous congestion** and **contusion**, there is also **proctorrhagia** of hemorrhoidal origin in varying quantities.

Collinsonia canadensis

This remedy is suitable for **hemorrhoids which tend to bleed**, specially in **constipated individuals** who produce large stools which are difficult to expel.

Prescribe twenty drops of *Collinsonia 3X* or *6X*, diluted in a little pure water, two to four times a day; this medicine may be mixed with equals parts of *Aesculus hippocastanum*.

Hamamelis virginiana

In experimental conditions, this substance causes **venous inflammatory phenomena** as well as **hemorrhages of black blood** and sensations of increasing pain or **bursting of the veins**, with aggravation with heat or with the slightest contact.

The dosage is identical to that of *Collinsonia canadensis* with which it may be combined; it may also be combined with *Aesculus hippocastanum*.

REMEDIES FOR HEMORRHOIDAL THROMBOPHLEBITIS

Faced with a painful acute attack of hemorrhoidal thrombophlebitis, the homeopath should immediately think of three remedies: *Arnica* (already mentioned), *Lachesis mutus*, and *Muriaticum acidum*.

Lachesis mutus

This remedy is suitable for **purplish, prolapsed hemorrhoids**, with **contact hyperesthesia**, throbbing pain, or the sensation of constriction in the anus. They are **relieved by bleeding** and aggravated by heat.

Muriaticum acidum

This remedy is used for **swollen, dark blue, bulging,** turgescent and hyperalgesic **hemorrhoids**; the patient cannot bear the slightest contact.

These three remedies, *Arnica, Lachesis,* and *Muriaticum acidum*, have pathogenic symptoms which are similar on the whole to the reactive clinical modalities of patients suffering from hemorrhoidal thrombosis. They are prescribed in turn, every hour or every two hours, five pellets in 9C, with an increased interval between doses as the severity of the symptoms diminishes.

REMEDIES FOR PRURITIC HEMORRHOIDS

Fluoricum acidum

This remedy is indicated if the hemorrhoids are **pruritic**, whether bleeding or not, especially if there is the notion of varices with heaviness in the lower limbs, on the condition that the characteristic modalities of **improvement by cold and/or cool showers** and aggravation with heat are present.

Paeonia officinalis

This remedy is prescribed for **painful, inflammatory hemorrhoids** which are very sensitive to the touch, with intense anal pain during or after defecation. **Pruritus is intense** with scratching and oozing.

Prescribe twenty drops of *Paeonia officinalis 3X* or *6X*, three or four times a day, diluted in a little pure water.

Ratanhia

The pathogenetic symptoms of this pharmacodynamic substance are scarcely different from those of *Paeonia officinalis*. The dosage is ideintical.

When it is difficult to individualize the remedies for bleeding and/or pruritus, it is advisable to prescribe "*Sepia composé*", a complex formula:

Sepia 3C
Aloe socotrina 3C
Arnica montana 3C
Sanguinaria canadensis 3C
Collinsonia canadensis 3C
Paeonia officinalis 3C
Aesculus hippocastanum 3X
Hamamelis virginiana 3X
} ana q.s. to 60 ml

This formula is delivered in the form of oral drops, tubes of pellets, and tablets. It is generally prescribed in a dosage of twenty drops two to four times a day.

HYGIENE AND DIETARY CARE

In a period of acute development, spices should be cut from the diet, as well as alcoholic beverages; light meals, plentiful soft drinks, and moderate exercise are advised.

There must be strict local hygiene: washing after every bowel movement and a sitz bath in cool water once or twice a day.

Ointments and suppositories have both a decongestant and a lubricating action to facilitate the expulsion of stools. The following medicines are also advised:
- *Aesculus composé suppositories* (2 or 3 every 24 hours);
- *Pommade Aesculus composé* (for local applications after each bowel movement or each wash);
- *Pommade Ratanhia* (in the case of pruritus).

INDEX

TABLE OF CONTENTS

Achevé d'imprimer par
l'Imprimerie Vasti-Dumas - 42010 Saint-Etienne
Dépôt légal : décembre 2009
N° d'imprimeur : V003542/00

Imprimé en France